DREAMS

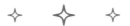

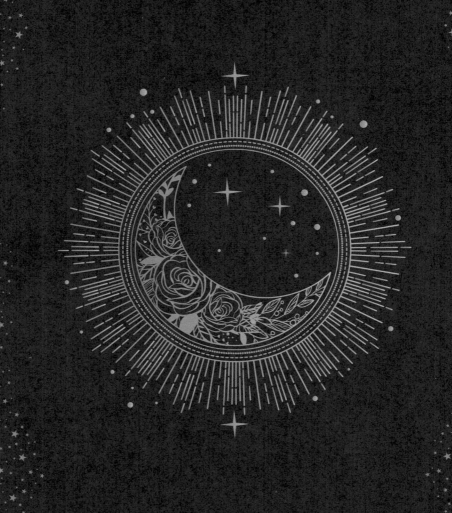

✦ DREAMS ✦

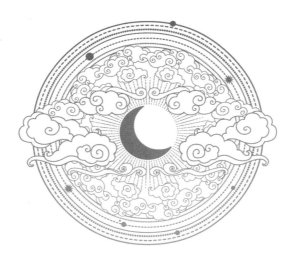

TOOLS FOR HARNESSING THE POWER
OF THE SUBCONSCIOUS

A Guide to Unlocking the Secrets of Your Personal Dream World

DR. FIONA STARR

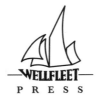

—WELLFLEET—
P R E S S

Inspiring | Educating | Creating | Entertaining

Brimming with creative inspiration, how-to projects, and useful
information to enrich your everyday life, Quarto Knows is a favorite
destination for those pursuing their interests and passions. Visit our
site and dig deeper with our books into your area of interest:
Quarto Creates, Quarto Cooks, Quarto Homes, Quarto Lives,
Quarto Drives, Quarto Explores, Quarto Gifts, or Quarto Kids.

Copyright © 2021 Quarto Publishing plc,
an imprint of The Quarto Group

This edition published in 2021 by Wellfleet Press,
an imprint of The Quarto Group,
142 West 36th Street, 4th Floor,
New York, NY 10018, USA
T (212) 779-4972 F (212) 779-6058
www.QuartoKnows.com

Conceived, edited, and designed by
Quarto Publishing plc,
6 Blundell Street, London, N7 9BH, UK.
QUAR: 341239

Wellfleet titles are also available at discount for
retail, wholesale, promotional, and bulk purchase.
For details, contact the Special Sales Manager by
email at specialsales@quarto.com or by mail at
The Quarto Group, Attn: Special Sales Manager,
100 Cummings Center Suite 265D, Beverly, MA 01915 USA.

10 9 8 7 6 5 4 3 2 1

ISBN: 978-1-57715-239-2

Library of Congress Control Number: 2021934633

Printed in China

CONTENTS

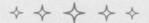

THE POWER OF DREAMS

Human beings have long been fascinated by dreams and their meanings. What are these images that inhabit our minds as we sleep? Thinkers and mystics have pondered their significance for thousands of years. While there is no single explanation as to why we dream, it is clear that the symbols, colors, settings, and emotions experienced are both universal and have a direct bearing on individual lives. Dreams help to guide us on journeys of self-discovery, the psychotherapist Carl Jung maintained.

The Dreams Box takes a closer look at the journeys we take while we sleep and offers guidance on how to understand your personal dream experiences. The first chapter looks at the ways in which dreams have been interpreted by different cultures over the centuries and considers how ancient people may have used dreams to shape their lives. It also introduces the theories of twenty-first-century psychologists Sigmund Freud and Carl Jung and goes on to examine the impact their works have had on modern-day dream interpretations.

Taking a more scientific view of what happens when we turn out the lights at night, the second chapter offers an overview of our sleep cycles and the influence they can have on our dreams.

Discover how to get the right kind of sleep to encourage dreaming—and even how to banish bad dreams. There is advice on keeping a dream record and instruction on taking those first important steps toward interpreting your dreams for yourself.

At the heart of the book, Unlock Your Dreams features a directory of dream archetypes and their various meanings. From the different people and animals that might appear in our dreams, through the familiar places and objects we encounter every day, to the significance of dominant colors, here are more than one hundred common dream symbols, each listed with its possible interpretations.

DREAM CARDS

The Dreams Box comes complete with a pack of thirty-six cards, each one representing an archetype in the directory section of the book. The cards can be used for guidance when interpreting the themes that take shape in your dreams. As well as using the cards to make sense of the dreams you have, you can use them to reinforce positive messages while repeling dreams with a negative edge. You will find instructions on using the cards on various pages in the chapters that follow.

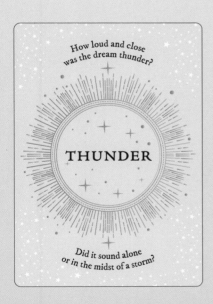

How loud and close was the dream thunder?

THUNDER

Did it sound alone or in the midst of a storm?

PLUS POINTS

- Close thunder traditionally signifies a trading victory, a successful harvest, or a happy marriage.
- Loud dream thunder also suggests that a frightening problem will soon be solved.

NEGATIVE IMPLICATIONS

- Distant dream thunder may represent a problem still "rumbling on."
- Thunder without a storm may warn that you need to make an imminent life change.

COUNTERBALANCE CARD: OCEAN

HEALING MESSAGE

Thunder was once thought to be the voice of the gods. In dreams it can be a clarion call to take action. *Examine pressing problems or decisions, and take steps to resolve them as soon as possible.*

The front of each card offers key questions about the dream you have had. On the back you will find both the plus points and the negative implications of the archetype. For the negatives, there is also a suggestion for a "counterbalance" card. Finally comes a healing message—a word of advice on how to react when this archetype features in your dreams.

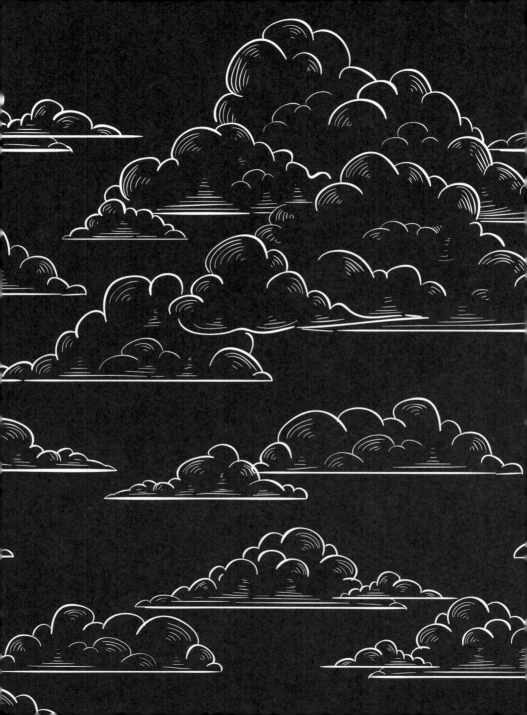

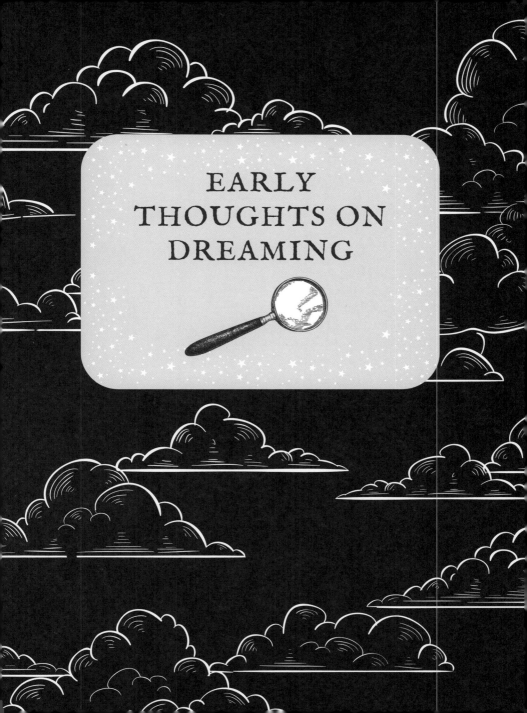

EARLY THOUGHTS ON DREAMING

GUIDANCE FROM THE GODS

While asleep, we lose consciousness and abandon control of our movements and thoughts. So who is directing the magical world of our dreams? The earliest dream interpreters believed that dreams were a means of communication with the gods.

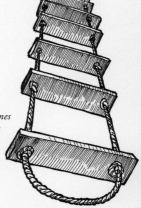

Ancient writings, such as Homer's epic poem *The Iliad*, where Zeus, the king of the gods, sends a message to the Greek commander Agamemnon, reflect this belief in a supernatural influence. Dreams were also thought to be signals. The Greek philosopher Socrates' decision to pursue music and the arts was said to have come to him in a dream.

Right: In the Bible, Jacob's ladder—sometimes staircase—symbolizes a connection between Heaven and Earth.

RELIGIOUS REVELATIONS

Throughout the Bible, God speaks to his prophets and disciples in dreams and visions. Perhaps the best known Old Testament dream is Jacob's dream of a ladder resting on top of Earth and reaching up to the heavens, channeling messages between God's angels and the planet below.

Dreams are significant in Islam as well. The prophet Muhammad, the founder of Islam, is said to have become aware of much of the Koran's contents from a dream. He was also well known for interpreting the dreams of his disciples.

A long Buddhist tradition of dream interpretation originates from India. The Buddha's mother had a dream in which a tiny white elephant entered her womb. Brahmins claimed that this dream predicted the birth of a great ruler.

For Zoroastrians, dreams are linked with their time of occurrence, so that a dream's place within the monthly cycle will affect its interpretation.

A HEALING ROLE

In both ancient Egypt and ancient Greece, people believed also that dreams have curative powers. Those in need of healing would sleep in temples for long periods of time in the hope of experiencing a dream that would forecast recovery.

Hippocrates (c. 460–375 BCE)—the founder of modern medicine—believed in using dreams as diagnostic tools. Other Greek thinkers also subscribed to this theory; as a result, many ancient Greeks were medically treated based on dreams that featured ailing parts of their bodies. Plato (c. 428–348 BCE) was especially interested in the influence of dreams on a person's mental and physical life. He believed that dreamed messages could signal how people should lead their lives.

For the Greek philosopher Aristotle (384–322 BCE), dreams were usually not prophetic; rather, they related to memories of the dreamer's waking day. Aristotle also wrote of dreams being "ignited" by the human senses. If a person became very hot when sleeping, for example, he or she might dream about heat or fire. Aristotle thought that metaphor was crucial in dream analysis. He suggested that dream images were not simply reflections of the waking world but metaphors for other images and situations.

SYMBOLIC MEANINGS

Aristotle's thinking forms the basis of modern dream analysis and is reflected in an early five-volume reference work on dreams, the Roman scholar Artemidorus' Oneirocritica *("The Interpretation of Dreams"), compiled around 150 CE. In this work, he espoused the theory that dreams were rooted in the dreamer's waking world. When a dream was interpreted, therefore, the dreamer's social status, place of work, and mental and physical condition should all be considered when attempting to decipher its content and meaning—a process used for dream interpretation today.*

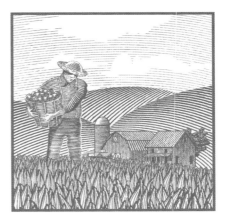

Artemidorus' book explains dreams featuring snakes and crocodiles, and activities including hunting, farming, and war.

HEALING THE SOUL

There is a long tradition of dream analysis in Western countries, particularly among the Native tribes of North America. Dream interpretation within other world cultures, such as those of Southeast Asia and Australia, is equally rich, and often markedly different.

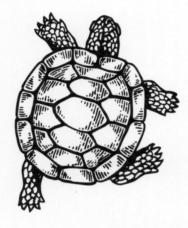

Left: Native American spiritual guides often take the form of a creature, such as a turtle, a deer, a wolf, or a raven.

For Native Americans, dreams and their messages are ways of predicting and understanding events. In many Eastern traditions, it is widely accepted that dreamers can actually influence their dream worlds.

Eastern dream analysts believe that by taking control of their dream worlds, dreamers can pursue a path of personal growth and spiritual development. In contrast to most Western thinkers, some also maintain that the dreamer can remain conscious while dreaming. Moreover, it is this conscious dreaming that enables the dreamer to gain the greatest spiritual rewards.

Certain Eastern philosophers describe the process of sleeping as a preparation for death. Each time we sleep, we ready ourselves for the time when we must die. It is thus in the dreamer's interest to prepare for sleeping and dreaming in the calmest and most comfortable way possible.

INFLUENCING DREAMS

Different Native American tribes, who use a variety of techniques to induce the dream state and to interpret dreams, also share a profound belief in the ability of dreamers to influence their dreams. They believe the dreamer can will the occurrence of a specific type of dream by concentrating upon the desired themes in the pre-dream state. The dream that follows then serves as a guide to show the dreamer how he or she should act upon waking. Preparations for the desired dream include praying, meditating, and fasting. Spending time at a peaceful and secluded location is also seen as an important inducement for entering the dream state.

Native Americans also claim that they can encounter a spiritual guide in their dreams, who may then assist them in some capacity. This spirit helper, who can reappear repeatedly in dreams, may impart a specific piece of knowledge or skill within the dream, such as a way of understanding an object or an aspect of the animal kingdom.

EMBRACING THE POSITIVE

In the Malaysian jungle, the Senoi people have developed their own form of dream interpretation. They believe that dreams can be controlled and modified in a positive sense while they are occurring. Thus a dreamer facing danger should tackle it head on. If something good happens in the dream, the dreamer should approach and embrace it; if evil is told to the dreamer, he or she should refuse to listen.

In this way, Senoi interpretations are connected to the dreamer's emotional development. Learning to deal with dream fears, for example, can help the dreamer to

manage real fears; welcoming pleasure in dreams can engender positive attitudes during wakefulness. Dreaming is therefore a two-way process: just as our waking emotions affect our dreams, the reverse can also occur.

In the Australian Aboriginal tradition, the recounting of dreams is a frequent, shared experience. For some tribes, if a dream subverts the expectations of the community—say a man experiences a sexual encounter in a dream, with a woman who is not his wife—something in the dream is expected to intercede.

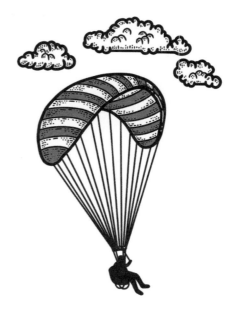

Right: Following the Senoi tradition, if you experience the pleasurable sensations of flying or swimming in a dream, you should relax and enjoy them fully.

THE ROLE OF THE UNCONSCIOUS

For modern psychologists, dreams are a principal access to the unconscious, reflecting—as the Malaysian Senoi people believe—real fears, repressed thoughts, feelings, and memories of which people may not be fully aware.

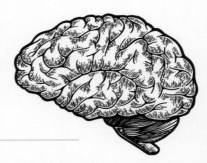

Psychologists believe that the unconscious influences emotions and behavior, but it cannot be accessed at will. Hypnosis, free association, and meditation may help to reach the unconscious, but the main means of access is through dreams.

Sigmund Freud pioneered the use of dreams as a way of connecting with a person's unconscious mind. His classic text *The Interpretation of Dreams* (1899) essentially summarized the study of dreams over the centuries and was extremely influential for two reasons: it established the concept that dreams and dreaming merited serious scientific study, and it addressed which questions to ask in relation to dream analysis.

Freud examined what the purpose of dreaming might be. He also considered how dreams might serve as vehicles for learning more about the workings of the human mind. He believed that the interpretation of dreams could have implications for the treatment of psychological problems, and that dreams could be used to monitor a patient's progress.

SEXUAL OR EROTIC DESIRES

Freud argued that the mind operates on both a primary and a secondary level. During the act of dreaming, a "primary process" occurs, in which the dreamer's unconscious desires or fears are turned into symbols, which then appear in the dream. The "secondary process" refers to the repression of these impulses and symbols by the conscious waking mind.

For Freud, dreams were generally intertwined with the dreamer's deepest desires and derived from emotions or events experienced in childhood. Freud also claimed that dreams were often the mind's way of expressing sexual or erotic desires, and that many dream images were symbols of sexuality. Thus, in his interpretations, long objects were often related to the penis, and certain fruits were associated with breasts.

WISDOM FROM WITHIN

While the Swiss psychologist Carl Jung collaborated with Freud for a time, he could not accept that dreams reflected only the dreamer's repressed desires, wish fulfillment or waking-life experiences. From his own research with many different individuals, he concluded that some dream symbols are innate in humans and shared across the world. Jung also believed that dreams play an important therapeutic role in the human psyche, connecting us to an internal higher source of wisdom, revealing the origin of current problems and supplying clues as to how they might be solved.

To aid interpretation, Freud had developed the idea of "free association," urging dreamers to focus on a recent dream, then to let the mind drift to trigger a hidden memory or emotion, which might shed light on a problem. Jung was concerned that this might lead dreamers too far from their dreams, causing them to lose touch with the important symbols within them. He developed a technique that he termed "direct association," which required dreamers to reflect on and make associations with specific aspects of the dream rather than dwelling on the dream as a whole.

REFLECTIONS OF WAKING LIFE

Unlike both Freud and Jung, Fritz Perls, a contemporary of Jung and founder of Gestalt therapy, contended that dreamers should conduct their own interpretations using their life experience, rather than relying on the guidance of a dream analyst. According to Perls, dream symbols are both projections of the dreamer's world and reflect the way the dreamer wants to lead his or her life. While Perls believed that dream symbols might also express deep-seated, unacknowledged elements of the dreamer's psychology, he maintained that dreams are purely reflections of the dreamer's waking life.

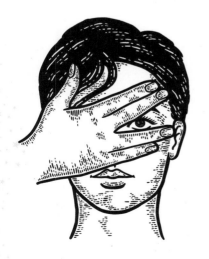

Left: A dream that features a human face may be linked with the dreamer's self-image, or with the image the dreamer projects to others.

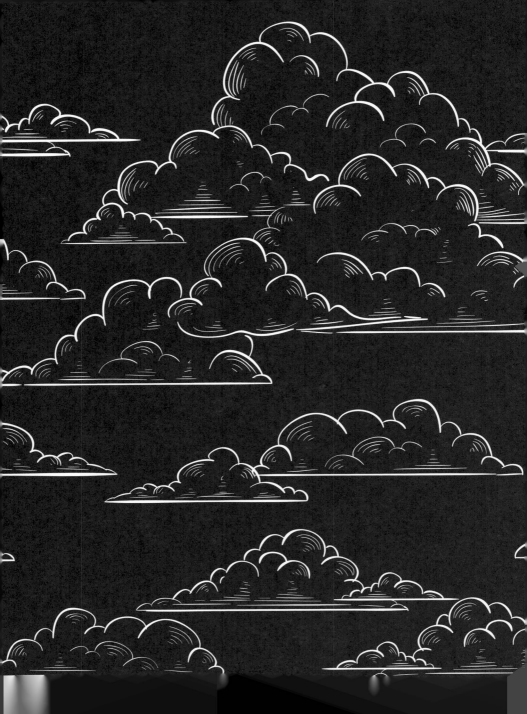

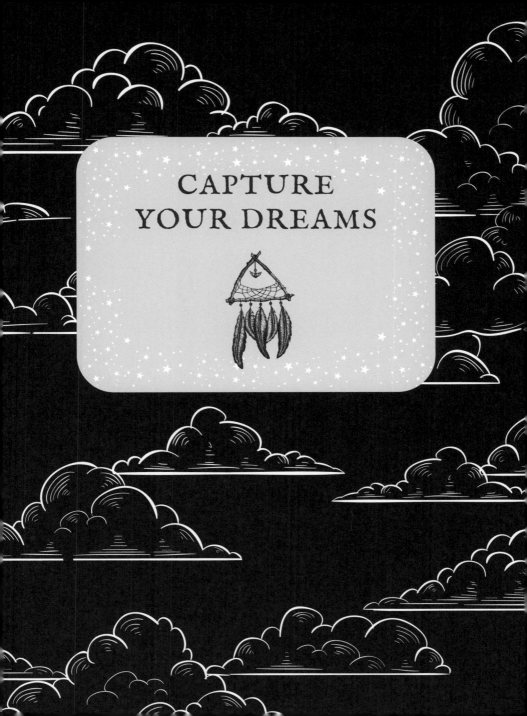

CAPTURE YOUR DREAMS

SLEEP'S MAGIC REALM

There are a number of ways to encourage dreaming and make it easier to study and interpret your dreams. It is important to get a good night's sleep and to dispel anxieties from your waking hours, which can interfere with sleeping and dreaming. Soothing scents, relaxation routines, and even perhaps your own "dream catcher" can all help. With practice and the help of the accompanying dream cards, you may find you can influence your own dreams. Carefully noting down details of your dreams will help you to identify symbols and emotions experienced while you sleep.

To dream, we must sleep, yet dreams do not occur throughout our sleeping hours. In the past fifty years, researchers have discovered that sleep has clearly differentiated stages, which can be determined by observing brainwaves and physiological activity.

During an average night's sleep, four phases of sleep occur. The cycle of movement from phase one through phase four usually happens about seven times a night. Each cycle lasts approximately ninety minutes.

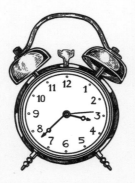

- ○ **Phase one**: The sleeper moves from wakefulness into sleep.
- ○ **Phase two**: This marks the beginning of actual sleep, where the sleeper is unaware of outside stimulation.
- ○ **Phase three**: There is a gradual continuation of the transition into deeper sleep.
- ○ **Phase four**: In this final phase, the sleeper sinks into an even deeper level of sleep. The sleeper breathes more rhythmically and deeply. Heart rate and blood pressure drop, the metabolism slows, and the electrical activity of the brain is different from its waking state.

THE DREAM PHASE

Phase four is also known as "rapid eye movement," or REM, sleep. This describes the process whereby the eyes dart rapidly from side to side under closed eyelids—and it marks the onset of dreaming. Dreams can happen in phases one, two, or three of the sleep cycle, but are less frequent and not as vivid as those occurring in REM sleep.

In 1953, the American physiologist Nathaniel Kleitman and his student Eugene Aserinsky discovered that if a sleeper was awakened while the electrical impulses of the brain exhibited certain rhythms, he or she reported dreaming at that time. The periods of brain activity and dreaming also corresponded with the occurrence of rapid eye movements. The rapid movements of the eye may actually represent the dreamer's observation of the events taking place in the dream. These discoveries marked the beginning of an intense period of study of dreaming and dream patterns.

WHY WE NEED REM SLEEP

Research has shown that newborn babies spend about half of their sleeping time in the REM state. Further, experiments have shown that people deprived of REM sleep become excessively sensitive, lose the ability to concentrate, and suffer poor recall.

In contrast, those deprived of non-REM sleep experience fewer and shorter-term difficulties. So it appears that in non-REM sleep, the body and mind are resting and regenerating. REM sleep, on the other hand, seems to be less physiologically but more psychologically important.

THE ROLE OF DREAMS

While a lack of REM sleep is harmful to our mental state, scientists continue to question the role of dreams. Are dreams a way to dispel unwanted waking experiences? Are they a means of processing daily events? Or are they an exercise for a part of the brain that remains dormant during waking hours?

As a result of studying dreams in laboratories, which allows for "on the spot" dream retrieval, scientists have discovered that the vast majority of dreams, including those experienced during an REM state, are mundane, highly realistic experiences, as opposed to bizarre, random occurrences. Further, dreams are also not usually faithful reproductions of memories; rather, they are novel experiences that have a thematic coherence, much like a story or novel. In most dreams, the dreamer experiences emotions appropriate to the particular situation in the dream.

While it seems likely that dreaming has a number of complex and interrelated physiological and psychological functions, one thing is clear. The dreams of each of us encapsulate aspects of our particular psyche and circumstances, including our situation, relationships, and experiences. An awareness of our dreams, therefore, can help us to increase our understanding of our thoughts and emotions.

SET YOUR DREAM SCENE

If you hope to have dreams to analyze, it is important to get a good night's sleep. Anxieties from your waking hours can inhibit the process of sleeping and dreaming. The following methods of preparation for sleep and dreaming are based on documented research and on individual experience.

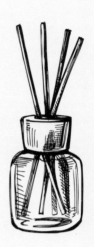

GETTING READY FOR NIGHTTIME REST

It is important not to sleep during the day if you want a good night's sleep. However tired you are, try to stay awake, so that your mind and body are aware of the differences between the waking zone and the sleeping zone. For consistently good sleep, go to bed at approximately the same time each night.

During the day, try to make sure you get enough exercise, eat balanced meals, and do not drink too much coffee or other caffeinated beverages, such as tea and cola drinks. Avoid alcohol and cigarettes for a few hours before going to bed, as both can disturb your sleep pattern.

SOOTHING SCENTS

To gain the most from your dreams, it is important to prepare for sleep calmly. Sometimes the associations of a particular smell can induce feelings of comfort. Add relaxing aromatherapy oils such as lavender, cypress, rose, marjoram, and chamomile to your bath. Vaporize the oil, or massage it into the skin, using a carrier oil such as almond oil. Most health food stores and some drug stores sell essential oils, often recommended for sleep disorders. But be careful when choosing aromatherapy products; certain essential oils, for instance, cannot be used by pregnant women. It is best to consult a qualified aromatherapist.

LEARN TO RELAX

Relaxation is not a passive activity—it requires a combination of physical and mental techniques, and a determination to focus the entire body and mind. Most people can, nevertheless, find a method of physical and mental relaxation that works for them. Taking a warm bath can help you to relax and is usually most effective about half an hour before bed. A warm milky drink, a chamomile tea, or a herbal infusion at bedtime can also be helpful. Some people listen to calming music.

Visualization is another popular way of relaxing for sleep. This process involves conjuring up images that will promote positive feelings in general—a peaceful, restful place, for example—and empty the mind of troubled, distressing, or over-stimulating images. Because of its ability to reduce stress and aid in relaxation, visualization can be an effective aid to sleep.

Gentle muscle relaxation, deep breathing, meditation, or yoga exercises may help to prepare you for sleep as well. These methods can require a little practice, but in time they may become a beneficial aid—not just to help you sleep, but for your well-being in general.

If you have little success with sleep-inducing techniques, however, do not remain in bed tossing and turning. It is better to get up and spend some time away from the bedroom, relaxing or listening to music, before trying to get to sleep again. Watching television, reading a stimulating book, or taking a walk as a means of distraction when you cannot sleep may not be helpful, as such activities stimulate the mind and body and can inhibit relaxation, and thus sleep. And always be sure to switch off your phone, so that callers do not interfere with the process of relaxation.

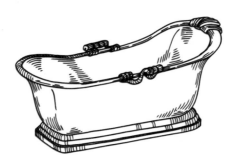

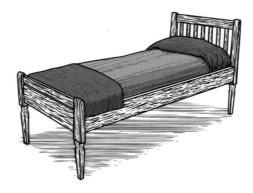

SOOTHING SURROUNDINGS

Since we spend approximately a third of our lives sleeping, where we sleep should be well designed for the purpose. The room should be peaceful and uncluttered, preferably without a television or any kind of phone. It should also be well aired, and neither too hot nor too cold—the recommended temperature is 65°F. If the atmosphere feels too dry or too stuffy, increase the humidity by placing bowls of water around the room, or damp towels over a radiator, or invest in an air humidifier.

Your bed is obviously the most important item in your sleeping room. You should buy the best mattress you can afford. It must be firm enough to support your back without sagging, especially as the muscles lose tension during REM sleep, leaving the ligaments to take the strain.

Lighting is significant when preparing your body for sleep. The brighter the lighting, the harder it is for your body to achieve a state of relaxation. Make full use of dimmer switches, low-voltage lamps, and gently colored lampshades. Make sure that your drapes are thick enough to block out street lights or sunshine—they can be lined, if necessary, with light-resistant fabric.

Pillows should be soft and comfortable, but firm enough to support your neck. It does not matter if they are filled with synthetic materials or down; allergy sufferers, however, should avoid feathers. The pillow should support your head rather than raise it.

BLOCKING BAD DREAMS

Hanging a colorful "dream catcher" over your bed can help to protect you from negative dreams. Legendary in the culture of Native Americans, this spiritual symbol was conceived by an elder of the Anishnabe tribe, who described a vision he had of a spiderweb, located inside a hoop, with a feather and a bead attached. These would hold on to positive dreams, his vision told him, while letting negative dreams pass through. Thus the first dream catchers were made, using willow, the feathers of an owl, and a bead or stone.

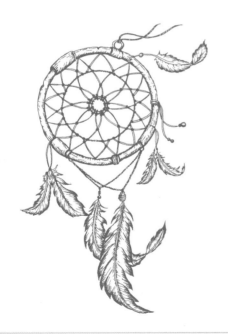

The dream catcher is placed above a sleeping area, in a position where it can attract the first rays of the morning light. According to Native American tradition, certain dreams are intended for particular people, conveying messages that are relevant only to them. The dream catcher cannot prevent these dreams from reaching the designated recipient; they will always pass through the web, and the dreamer must dream their important symbols or messages.

The dream catcher can, however, block the free-floating bad dreams that are believed to inhabit the night sky. In the absence of dream catchers, these bad dreams drift unchecked and can visit sleepers, troubling them. The dream catcher holds back the bad dreams, which are then destroyed by the rays of the early morning sun.

A good dream is believed to follow the bead or stone into the center of the web, and then into the mind of the person sleeping beneath the dream catcher. The good dreams are allowed to move back and forth through the center of the dream catcher, and can thus be dreamed again, by the same person or by other dreamers.

RECORD YOUR DREAMS

Although we cannot always remember our dreams, they often leave behind feelings that remain with us during our waking hours. Recording our dreams can help us remember them, and can thus help identify the sources of these lingering emotions.

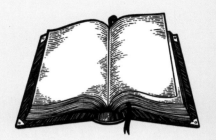

START A DREAM DIARY

Most dream analysts recommend recording the contents of your dreams in a dream diary. In addition to helping you recall the dream's details, the diary will provide a record for study, enabling you to identify patterns and themes within your dreams.

A psychological and practical commitment to the process of recording your dreams is the first step on the path to interpretation.

FIRST STEPS TO DREAM INTERPRETATION

When you note down your reactions to the dream (interpretation page, see opposite), list them as positive or negative messages, and describe how they made you feel. Record colors and whether they are associated with specific objects or persons. The chapter that follows will help you to interpret their meaning. Use them as a basis for your analysis. Be sure to note any events from the previous day that may have influenced your dream. It can also be helpful to write down what you were thinking about just prior to falling asleep.

Read back over the contents of your diary occasionally; you may notice recurring themes in your dreams. It can be useful to add an overall analysis page to your diary from time to time, in order to tie recent themes together.

USING DREAM CARDS

The accompanying dream cards represent the thirty-six most universal dream images. Find those that most closely match your dream experience and use their wisdom, too, to help you understand its meaning. They clearly indicate positive and negative implications and can help to explain the psychological significance of these dream events. Each card also indicates a complementary card that can counterbalance any negative influences.

Lay out recurring images on your bedside table. Carefully read their messages and consider their meanings in your daily life. To reinforce a positive message, carry a significant card with you throughout the day. Repel negative dreams at night by placing both the relevant card and its counterbalance card under your pillow.

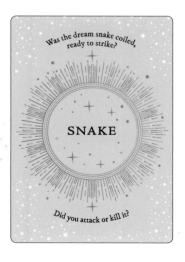

KEEPING A DREAM DIARY

○ *Choose a method that you find practical to maintain. Your diary can take any form. Most people keep a notebook and a flashlight by their beds, but an audio diary works as well.*

○ *Record your dream before getting out of bed, as activity can cause the memory to fade.*

○ *Make brief outline notes but be sure to mention even seemingly trivial or obscure aspects of the dream, as these can contain clues to its meaning.*

○ *While the dream is still fresh in your mind, record it in full. A large diary or exercise book is recommended.*

○ *Write down the details of the dream on the left-hand page (the recollection page) and any thoughts and associations on the right-hand side (the interpretation page).*

○ *Date your dream; this may be relevant to its meaning. It might occur on a significant anniversary or when a deadline is looming, and this will help you put the dream into context.*

○ *Record events, scene by scene, just as they unfold in your dream. Adding diagrams and pictures may help impress them on your mind.*

TAKING CONTROL

We think of dreaming as an unconscious activity,
but in some dreams we may be fully aware of what
we are dreaming and may also have the ability
to control the outcome of a dream.

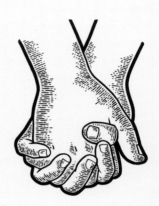

Modern dream experts call this "lucid"
dreaming—a term coined in 1913 by
Dutch physician Willem van Eeden, who
reported experiencing mental arousal and
a high state of awareness during his dreams.
Though lucid dreams are rare for most
people, it is possible to teach yourself to
dream lucidly.

*Above: Lucid dreaming can help you find
solutions to conflicts in your waking life—in
relationships, for example.*

A LONG EASTERN TRADITION

While less common in the West, the notion
that we can take control of our dreams and
thereby steer our destiny is common in the
East, and examples have been documented
for centuries in many different cultures. In
some of the world's main religions, lucid
dreaming has mystical associations. In the
Hindu and Buddhist traditions, certain
people are thought to have the ability to
remain conscious while dreaming. Tibetan
Buddhists believe that the very purpose of
dreaming is to allow the conscious mind to
influence and control the unconscious.

DIRECTING THE DREAM

The unique quality of lucid dreams means
that they are usually remembered. The lucid
part of the dream reflects the clarity of the
dreamer's level of consciousness rather than
the vividness of the dream. In the middle of
such a dream, the dreamer becomes aware
that he or she is dreaming, and the dream
becomes more realistic as this realization
occurs. A dreamer who can retain this state
of consciousness may then be able to
influence the events in the dream.

TEACH YOURSELF TO DREAM LUCIDLY

Some people report having had lucid dreams spontaneously, but for most of us some training is needed. In order to dream lucidly, you must first be able to remember your dreams. As you gain familiarity with dream symbols and with recurrent dream themes, it will become easier to recognize the point in your sleep cycle when dreaming is occurring.

You are more likely to experience a lucid dream when you have had a good sleep. Performing a few relaxation techniques can help you to prepare for lucid dreaming. It can also be useful to recite to yourself that when

you dream in the night, you will dream lucidly and will be aware that you are experiencing a dream.

Keeping a dream diary (see page 25) is another way to induce your mind to engage in lucid dreams. The records in your diary will help you to recognize familiar images and dream scenarios, so that when they recur, you may become consciously aware that your mind has entered the dream state.

DREAM CARD HELP FOR LUCID DREAMING

If certain images frequently recur, use the accompanying dream cards to identify a pattern and also to influence your dreams. For instance, fire—a symbol of light, spirituality, and inner power—is also linked with extreme emotions. You may need to change or purge some aspect of your life. Place the Fire card under your pillow to help you take charge of events in your fire dream, and to face up to responsibilities and decisions in your life. If your fire dream suggests obstacles to be overcome, place the counterbalancing Sky card under your pillow, too, to help clear the way.

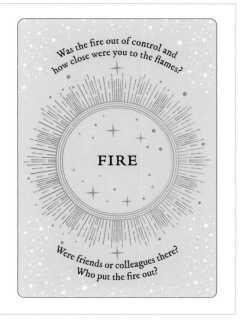

Was the fire out of control and how close were you to the flames?

FIRE

Were friends or colleagues there? Who put the fire out?

GO WITH THE FLOW

When you sense that you are moving from a period of ordinary dreaming to lucid dreaming, it is important to relax. If you can manage not to focus on your conscious mind, but to let yourself "go with the flow," you are likely to be able to continue sleeping and dreaming as you desire. If you can remain in a lucid state, you may be able to reach a new level of consciousness. The more often this happens, the longer the lucidity will last, and the easier it should be to achieve this state on your next attempt.

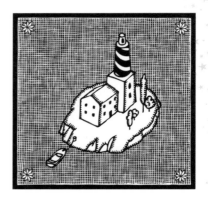

PRACTICE DEEP RELAXATION

Meditation, self-hypnosis, and autosuggestion can all result in a state of consciousness similar to lucid dreaming. These techniques—which also assist in relaxation, and can thus encourage a full night's sleep—can help give you a sense of what lucid dreaming is like. They can be self-taught, but are more likely to be successful when learned with the help of a reputable practitioner.

If successful, these techniques will bring about a state of deep relaxation by focusing your mind on breathing, directing it to ignore the continuous interior flow of dialogue, thoughts, and images, and quietly repeating a certain phrase, or mantra.

FANTASY ISLANDS

Once you have achieved a state of complete mental and physical calm, you can allow yourself to introduce controlled images into your mind. These visualizations may consist of a special serene location that you visited in your waking life, or a fantasy place unique to you. Upon reaching this place, spend some imaginary time there relaxing. As with any relaxation technique, visualization does not come magically, and can require persistence to make it work. The more often you practice, the easier it will become to achieve this special level of consciousness.

You can also use the achievement of a state of deep relaxation to visualize a difficult situation at work, or within your family. Imagine yourself overcoming this challenge—and the outcome of the situation. As with lucid dreaming, this process can help you resolve difficulties in your waking life.

LUCID SOLUTIONS

Learning to dream lucidly can be beneficial; no harmful effects have been reported. In fact, a lucid dream can seem less threatening than an ordinary dream, because you feel that you possess some control over it. If something frightening enters the dream, you can simply make it go away. Similarly, if a work colleague who is causing you problems appears, you can direct yourself to resolve the situation within the dream.

There are, however, mixed opinions about the value of lucid dreaming. Some argue that allowing our consciousness to enter the dream state and exert control over it can be a positive experience, while others consider lucid dreaming to go against the primary function of ordinary dreaming—the expression of the unconscious mind, free from interference.

MEASURING DREAM TIME

Sleep researchers have used lucid dreams to try to establish how much time a dream actually occupies. Do dreams condense time, as is widely believed, or do dream events occupy a real time interval? A team of researchers at Stanford University, in California, asked lucid dreamers to carry out previously agreed eye movements to indicate their progression through a predetermined sequence of dream events. They concluded that dream time approximates to real time. Further, they found evidence that dreams may omit unnecessary periods of time that happened in our waking lives, but were not needed in our dreams.

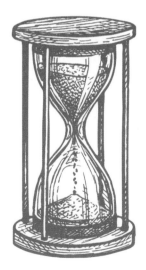

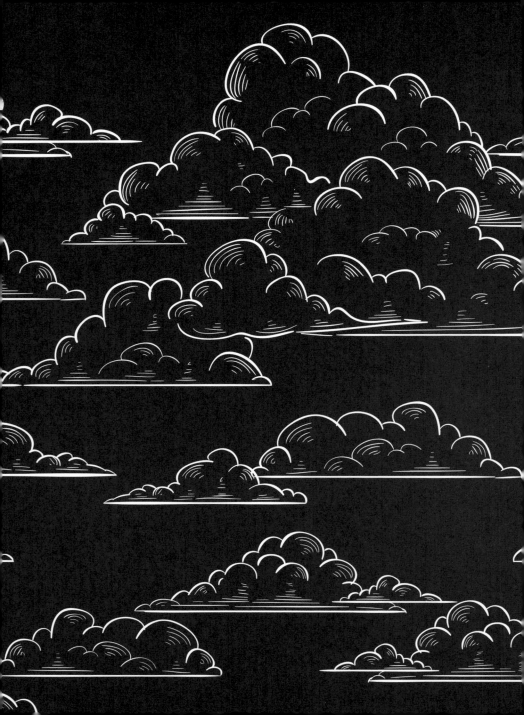

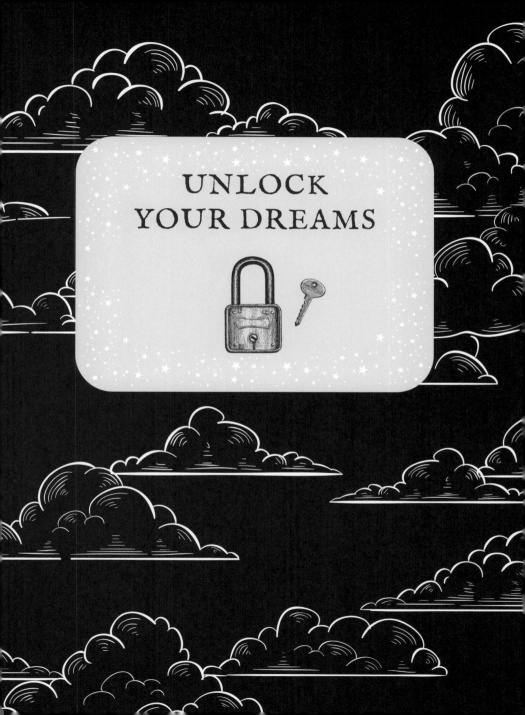

RECURRENT THEMES

Certain themes appear consistently in people's dreams, and can be identified by the images, or symbols, that occur within them. Thus, careful consideration of the meaning of each symbol in a dream will help uncover its meaning. The feelings experienced by the dreamer in a dream can also provide clues to its meaning. This is healing knowledge that can help resolve current anxieties and problems, and direct future actions.

DECODE THE SYMBOLS

Sigmund Freud pioneered the use of dreams as a way of connecting with the unconscious, and he established the concept that dreaming merited scientific study. He maintained that the function of dream symbols was to allow humans to sleep while permitting the id—the part of the mind that contains our most primitive instincts—to express animalistic desires. By the 1920s, many scientists and psychologists disagreed with his theory. In their view, dreams did not unlock our repressed, hidden desires; rather, they were reflections of the dreamer's waking life.

JUNGIAN ARCHETYPES

While Carl Jung agreed that dreams generally represent the dreamer's unconscious mind, he questioned whether dreams were solely the product of the dreamer's personal experiences, and so began to look for identical themes in the dreams of different individuals. He discovered notable similarities between the dream imagery, associations, and delusions of a broad range of his psychotic patients. Having a keen interest in mythology, world religions, and the occult, he also noticed associations between key elements of those studies and recurrent themes in people's dreams.

Jung believed that these common themes derived from a shared body of historical and cultural myths and stories throughout the world. He concluded that there must exist some form of "collective unconscious," an inborn store of information, linked with a human tendency to organize and interpret experiences in similar ways regardless of culture and background. In this way, Jung introduced the concept of a universal "archetype"—an innate idea or pattern that could emerge within dreams in the form of a basic symbol or image.

UNIVERSAL MEANING

Jung described archetypes as primeval images and ideas that contain meaning for all people at all times. He claimed they were not only expressed in dreams, but also in forms of folklore such as fairy tales and legends.

The archetypes are personalized according to each individual's experience, but readily recognizable archetypal figures and events include the mother, dream animals, and death. According to Jung, dream symbols can only be properly understood when related to their archetypal meanings. To interpret dreams, it is essential to consider what each archetype might represent to the dreamer.

AN ALMOST RELIGIOUS FUNCTION

In his quest to unravel the meanings of dreams, Jung analyzed every dream occurrence in three distinct contexts: the personal, the cultural, and the archetypal. He believed that dreams exercised an almost religious function and could contribute to a process that points individuals in the direction of spiritual enlightenment. For Jung, therefore, the dream was not just a reflection of repressed desires or a form of wish fulfillment, but also a conduit through which people could make a connection with their "higher" or wiser selves. The dream could also reveal the roots of a person's present problems, and it might contain clues about how to solve them.

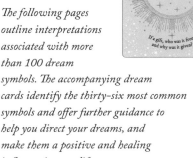

YOUR HEALING GUIDE

The following pages outline interpretations associated with more than 100 dream symbols. The accompanying dream cards identify the thirty-six most common symbols and offer further guidance to help you direct your dreams, and make them a positive and healing influence in your life.

SPIRITUAL GROWTH

Jung chose the basement of a beautiful house as his image of the place that most humans inhabit. The whole house, with its fascinating and diverse rooms, represents the enormous potential for creative and spiritual growth possessed by all human beings. Many of us, however, confine ourselves to the basement, and do not realize our potential.

For Jung, dreams were a means of gaining access to the other rooms of the house, and dream interpretation was the means of exploration. The more people understood about dreams and their layers of meaning, the more they would understand various aspects of their personal and emotional lives.

ACCESSING YOUR UNCONSCIOUS

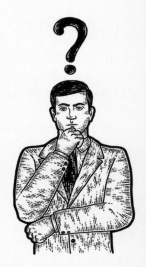

Thanks to the work of Jung and Freud, we understand that dreams reflect our emotions, aspirations, and deepest thoughts and fears. In a way that is not fully understood, each day of our waking lives our minds unconsciously absorb millions of sights and sounds, which dreams then render back, often curiously transformed.

Making sense of these messages and getting in touch with our unconscious are important for our psychological health. A fear can thus be acknowledged and tackled by day. Anger and ill-feeling can be recognized and resolved. Troubling memories can be unearthed, re-examined, and neutralized. The set of cards that accompany this book can help you to do this. For example, being chased is frightening in a dream. With the help of the "chasing" dream card, you will quickly uncover the implications, and understand if this is a real or perceived threat. As importantly, the card offers a "healing message," which will help you to control and direct future "chasing" dreams.

USING THE CARDS

Look through the pack carefully and pick out the cards that immediately resonate with your experience. Carefully read their message and look through the following pages to find more specific interpretations. If you feel any card is especially helpful, keep it with you and put it under your pillow at night. Add its suggested "counterbalance card" if you have been troubled by negative thoughts.

For further inspiration and to delve more deeply into your subconscious, think about any current fears or problems you are facing, particularly if they have surfaced in recent dreams. Then pick a card at random and see if its words can help you to find an answer.

BRIDGING THE GAP

Whether our dreams are simply projections of our own world, or whether they reflect broader cultural archetypes, as Jung believed, they are often far removed from reality. Yet, with effort and practice, we may be able to exert some control over them—to our benefit. For example, a dream of killing suggests some of the most intense feelings any of us will ever experience. It may represent

FREE ASSOCIATION

The dream cards can help you to access your unconscious during waking life. Freud developed the idea of free association, a technique involving three stages, which can be used in conjunction with the cards as follows:

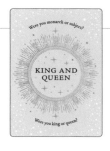

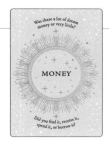

1 *In the first stage, focus on a recent dream. At this point, select a card that corresponds to any image in your dream and study the front of the card, focusing only on the word at its center.*

2 *In the second stage, allow your mind to drift and see what further images come to mind in association with the dream. At this point, writing down a list may help. If any other dream cards match your "association" list, pick them up, too.*

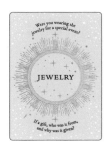

3 *Finally, in the third stage, you should examine the list and cards to establish their significance, and whether they prompt the recall of a forgotten memory or the surge of a particular emotion. It is here that the cards' healing messages may also help to resolve a current or deep-seated problem.*

Whether your dreams trouble or intrigue you, the book and cards are designed to bring fresh insights. Unlocking the coded messages of the night can undoubtedly help resolve both emotional and practical problems, heal the soul, and only enhance your waking life.

repressed fury, which must be more closely examined in daylight hours.

With the help of your "killing" dream card—and perhaps with that card and its counterbalancing "ocean" card tucked under your pillow—you can attempt a dream resolution. (See also "Taking Control," pages 26–29). If there is an enemy, deflect the ill-feeling; offer an olive branch in your dream or similar symbol of peace. Or examine whether your dream might have a positive interpretation—perhaps this "killing" is putting an end to some unpleasant episode. Reflect on a scene of calm, blue-green water to induce a sense of peace.

DREAM FIGURES AND FEATURES

Familiar characters in our dreams are often associated with those who inhabit our waking lives; they may also signify different aspects of our personalities. Dreams involving the human body are usually about our own body, and they tend to reflect our feelings about it, so may be associated with self-esteem.

ARCHETYPES

ASSOCIATED CARDS

○ Wedding

○ Parents

○ King and Queen

○ Face

○ Eyes

○ Hair

○ Teeth

○ Blood

BRIDE AND GROOM

A wedding couple appearing in a dream is often regarded as a symbol of union. Depending on the circumstances of the dream event, the two figures can express a state of harmony or, conversely, opposition prevailing in differing parts of the psyche. A dream bride or groom appearing alone can also represent an external union between the dreamer and another person.

YOUR PLACE IN THE DREAM Your role at the wedding is perhaps the most crucial factor to consider, particularly if you were the bride or groom, or a member of the wedding party. The atmosphere at the wedding ceremony can also be telling. Was it a joyful occasion, or was it shrouded in sadness or fear?

DREAM DESIRES A dream involving a wedding couple may be mere wish fulfillment, especially if you were the bride or groom. If the bride or groom were going off on a honeymoon, this may represent the anticipation of an imminent pleasurable event. Or you may be envious. Some interpreters believe that seeing a bride or groom in a dream can signify jealousy or rivalry.

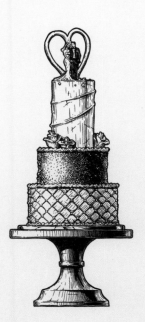

BRIDE OR GROOM? A woman's dream of a groom suggests a need to get in touch with the masculine side of her personality. Similarly, when a man dreams of a bride, he may need to listen to his feminine side. If the bride or groom in your dream was your current partner, you may need reaffirmation of his or her love.

YOUR RELATIONSHIPS A dream of a wedding can suggest commitment to a current relationship and a desire for it to last. Alternatively, the dream may signal a fear of commitment. Consider the emotional state of the dream bride and groom. Were they radiant and excited, or fearful and unhappy?

MOTHER AND FATHER

Dreams about parents may simply express feelings and memories about these closest of all relatives. The dream father can symbolize a strong moral conscience; childhood experiences of the father as a powerful guide and judge may resonate in the dreamer's mind. The dream mother can reflect your feelings about the powerful mother-child relationship.

PARENTAL BONDS Dreams about fathers and mothers are traditionally interpreted as signs of parental love. A dream father may represent a figure of playfulness and affection. A dream mother may symbolize the warmth and closeness of your relationship; or, the presence of the mother figure may indicate a need to break away from over-attachment.

CRYING MOTHER A dream of your mother in tears can be linked with your own concerns about a problem in your waking life. Some analysts believe that a crying mother signifies trouble ahead.

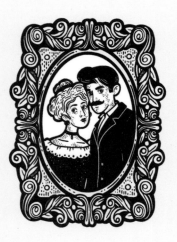

BENEVOLENT FATHER The appearance of a benevolent father in a dream is sometimes linked with interests or hobbies in which you show only a passing interest, and which you do not intend to pursue seriously. Such a dream may be a signal for you to broaden your horizons and find a new project to take on.

DISCIPLINE Dreaming of being disciplined by your parents signifies feelings of powerlessness. Think about how you might reclaim some control in your life without being too confrontational with others.

LYING A dream in which you lie to your parents may be a sign that you are about to complete a transaction, possibly in secret. A dream in which your parents lie to you suggests that you feel excluded from a social group.

PARENTAL ABANDONMENT Dreams in which one or both parents abandon you are usually linked with concerns about the solidity of your financial foundations. If your parent or parents return, your concern is probably unfounded. If not, this may be a signal that you need to face up to any financial problems in your waking life.

KINGS AND QUEENS

Dream kings and queens can symbolize the dreamer's father and mother. The remoteness and power of regal figures may represent the dreamer's true feelings about his or her parents or other authority figures. Dreaming about royalty can also reflect a desire for increased status or power. If you dream you are a monarch, try to recall how this position was attained, and how you treated your "royal court."

CHESS MOVES If your dream king and queen are chess pieces, think about their moves and whom they threaten. A king in check may be a sign that a female figure in your life is smothering your individuality. A threat to the queen may be a warning to be wary of overbearing males.

THE KING'S SEAT A dream in which a king is seated on a majestic throne may signify a suspicion that someone is cheating you in your waking life.

THE GRACIOUS QUEEN A dream queen waving at a crowd from a balcony can foretell the arrival of news from a distant location. If the dream queen was riding in an ornate carriage, this may be connected to a hidden desire for power or fame—a desire of which you are ashamed.

QUEEN OF CARDS If the queen appears as a symbol on a playing card, your dream may be connected to feelings of overconfidence or arrogance. It is worth thinking before you speak or act boldly—you may well regret any rash comments or deeds.

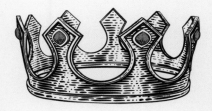

ROYAL CROWN A crown can symbolize a future prize that is currently just out of your grasp. However, a dream featuring the crowning of a king can be interpreted as a symbol that business or financial matters are proceeding according to plan.

HUMAN FACE

A dream that features a human face may be linked with the dreamer's self-image, or with the image the dreamer projects to others. The human face is usually the first and most significant part of a person's body to be noticed, and therefore conveys our image most powerfully to the outside world. The dream face can thus reflect how you wish to be seen.

REFLECTING REALITY If the face is bright and has clear, fresh skin, this could be you as you are—or as you would wish to be. A haggard face may signify that you are unhappy with your image in the eyes of others. The dream face can also reflect your daily routine in waking life. Was it showing the effects of a hectic schedule?

AGED FACE A wrinkled face may simply be a representation of an older person in your life. Such an image can also symbolize longevity and wisdom; your dream may be a sign that you are seeking guidance in your waking life.

FAMILIAR FACES A multitude of familiar faces may indicate a forthcoming celebration or social event—possibly one that you have already planned. Were they from the same family or group, or did they represent several different areas of your life?

A NOSE FOR FRIENDS A dream in which your nose is the focus can signify that you possess a greater social circle than you realize. Blowing your dream nose can foretell an increase in personal or family tasks that will bring satisfaction. A blocked nose can reveal that your plans face opposition.

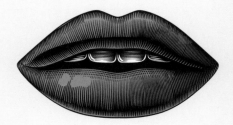

LIPS AND MOUTH Prominent lips on a dream face are generally interpreted as a symbol of the female genitalia. They may also signify the need to communicate more directly with persons close to you. Dream mouths may have a sexual meaning, too, but are also linked with nourishment. A smiling or frowning mouth can indicate how nurtured or loved you feel.

A MANLY BEARD Beards are often interpreted as symbols of masculinity but may also be connected to the female side of a man's character—especially if the mouth is visible.

EYES

In ancient times, the eyes were said to symbolize faith. They have also been called the windows of the soul, revealing the true nature of their owner's psyche. In dreams, the eye's ability to perceive was believed to mirror the dreamer's understanding of the world. Such interpretations persist today. Dream eyes are also believed to be a conduit to the future, with the capacity to predict events through clairvoyant vision.

PREDICTING MOOD The warmth or coldness of a dream eye expression may be linked with a dreamer's well-being. If the eyes are smiling, the dreamer may be experiencing—or about to enter—a period of contentment in waking life. Worried dream eyes may reveal the dreamer's fear of emotional or psychological isolation.

EYE INJURY OR DISEASE Dreaming of an eye injury or disease can indicate real fears concerning your reputation. Are you worried that someone is questioning your good character or plotting against you? Consider whether such a threat exists—and, if so, whether something can be done about it.

☞ **EYEBROWS AND LASHES** Dream eyebrows—especially shapely or attractive ones—can be symbols of dignity and honor, and may foretell the respect you will receive from an unexpected group of people. A dream of hair loss from the eyebrows can signify a loss of social standing. A dream featuring one or more eyelashes may be connected with a secret that was shared with you—possibly a revelation that would cause difficulties if it were passed on.

EYES IN ISOLATION Eyes that are disconnected from a face can denote an upturn in your financial situation. A floating eye or eyes may reveal a secret desire to take a risk in monetary matters. Extreme caution is needed with regards to any such venture.

EYE SHAPE The shape of dream eyes can be significant. If they are wide and open, this may represent innocence or childlike excitement. If they are narrow or closed, this may carry connotations of deceit.

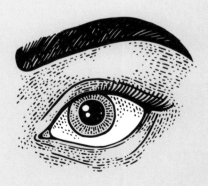

EARS, HAIR, AND TEETH

Dreams about ears are usually linked with listening, and can suggest that the dreamer should pay more heed to the words of others. They may also suggest a fear that in waking life someone is withholding important information from them. The condition of dream hair—whether healthy or in poor condition—is an indication of self-image. Teeth in dreams also often relate to feelings of self-worth.

BIG, SMALL, OR ANIMAL EARS The size of the dream ears can be significant. Exceptionally large ears can imply that assistance may come from an unexpected person, while small ears may suggest that you will discover that a colleague or friend has been untrue. Dreaming that you possess the ears of a strange or wild animal may also symbolize the fear that someone is deceiving you.

EAR WASHING A dream involving washing your ears may suggest that good news is on the way. If you washed your own ears, you may be the bearer of the news; if someone else washed them, the news may come from others.

PULLING EARS A dream in which your ear is pulled—or you pull someone else's ear—may signify a dispute in the workplace.

HAIR POWER Dream hair can be a symbol of sexuality. In men it is connected with virility; in women it is associated with attracting a partner. Dreams of perfumed hair may be associated with arrogance or vanity.

CUTTING AND COMBING Having your hair cut can signify success in a new undertaking. Cutting another's hair may be a warning to heed those who appear hostile toward you. Combing your own or other people's hair is related to successful problem solving.

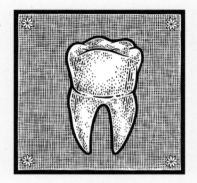

EXTRACTING TEETH A dream of pulling out one or more of your own teeth is thought to be a warning: do not act until you have considered a problem from all angles. An obstruction dislodged from the teeth can signify that a seemingly intractable problem might soon be solved. A more persistent blockage suggests the process could take longer.

TOOTHBRUSHING Cleaning teeth in a dream is often connected with the giving of money to friends or relations.

HANDS, LEGS, AND FEET

Dream hands often act as signposts for the dreamer in waking life. A delicate hand may indicate a particular direction, whereas a weathered hand may point an entirely different way. A dream involving legs can reflect the extent to which you feel supported by friends, colleagues, or family. Dream feet are thought to represent progress in the dreamer's life, especially if they are walking forward.

STROKING The caressing of hands in a dream usually implies friendship or romance —sometimes, even marriage. If you stroked another person's hand, consider their significance in your waking life.

WARNING Dirty dream hands can be a warning to curb bad behavior, or else others will think less of you.

DREAM DEXTERITY Were your dream hands easy or hard to manipulate? The dexterity of dream hands can be linked with personal matters. If hard, did you feel frustrated, or did you patiently persevere?

STRONG LEGS A dream featuring strong, healthy legs implies a sense of contentment both at home and at work. But if you had a wooden leg in your dream, you may feel overly reliant on some form of external assistance.

IRRITATION Itchy legs may be a sign that a worry about a current concern is a waste of your time and energy.

WALKING FEET A dream of many feet walking together is said to signify potential material loss. Such a dream could be a warning to attend to your financial situation.

FOOT STRENGTH The determination or strength of the dream feet may indicate how you are approaching a task. Will a present goal be a "walkover"—or will it require hard work?

BATHING FEET A dream of bathing your own feet, or someone else washing them, can mean that you have distanced yourself from everyday worries.

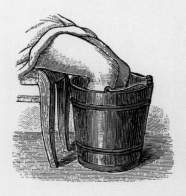

BREAST, SPINE, AND BUTTOCKS

Dreams about breasts are often sexual in nature. They can also relate to maternal feelings and relationships, and may denote a desire for psychological or emotional nourishment. The backbone in dreams may represent human will, and your capacity for determination, courage, and self-belief. Buttocks appear frequently in dreams. A dream of whipping them may reveal a conscious or unconscious sexual appetite.

MOTHER FIGURE Often connected with nature and growth, dream breasts can symbolize Mother Earth. They may signify that you are undergoing a period of personal development, spiritual enlightenment, or inner healing. The breasts may also represent an excessive attachment to a particular person, usually your mother or another maternal figure.

RESTING HEAD A dream of resting the head on someone's breast suggests the potential to form a new and long-lasting friendship.

BREAST SIZE Full dream breasts can be a sign of good times to come. Conversely, small or wrinkled breasts may foretell a future hardship of some kind.

SPINE SHAPE While a straight, strong spine in your dreams can signify inner strength, a curved spine may reveal a lack of will; it may imply a need to stand up for yourself at work or at home. The straightness of your dream spine can also reflect the degree to which you feel united with your unconscious.

KICKING BUTTOCKS A dream of kicking someone's buttocks can be a sign that you hope for promotion at work. Aiming to kick, but missing, may suggest that a project will fail unless you stick closely to your plan. Someone kicking your buttocks can signify that you are experiencing disapproval from some source.

SEX, SOCIAL EVENTS, OR SHAME If the dream is obviously sexual, whose buttocks were featured? Try to make a connection with your waking sexual desires. Dreaming of several pairs of buttocks can foretell pleasant social events ahead. Naked dream buttocks may also signify feelings of shame or guilt.

♉ ANIMAL BUTTOCKS The appearance of animal buttocks in a dream can be an omen of wealth of some kind.

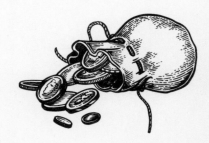

BLOOD

Often said to represent life itself, blood frequently appears in dreams and is related to personal strength and spiritual matters. Blood may also signify rejuvenation, which could take the form of physical recovery, emotional awakening, or spiritual rebirth. The deep red color of blood and its role as a life force are often linked with passion, love, or anger, too.

STRONG EMOTIONS A dream of rich crimson blood, flowing freely, can symbolize the dreamer's intense passion for a person or a situation. It can also suggest unconscious feelings of anger toward someone close to the dreamer in waking life.

NEW BLOOD A dream in which you are having a blood transfusion can indicate that you are on the verge of solving a current problem.

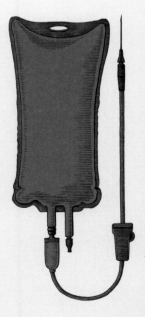

BLOOD LOSS The loss of blood generally refers to a deterioration of physical, spiritual, or moral strength. If the blood flowed from a wound, you should be wary of tentative work projects or business proposals.

FLOWING FREE Circulating blood in a dream can be an important symbol. If your dream blood moved through arteries or veins with ease, this may signify that you feel you are on the right life path. Any blockage could represent perceived obstacles to your life plan. A dream of gushing blood can mean that you feel drained in some way and are, perhaps, in need of greater personal fulfillment.

BLOOD STAINS Blood on your hands in a dream can relate to deep-seated guilt about an action or sphere of your life. Bloodstained clothes may be a sign that someone wishes to impede you at work or to hinder your ability to pursue a fulfilling career.

RITES, RITUALS, AND DEATH

Dreams involving the key stages of life often indicate beginnings or endings in areas of the dreamer's waking world. Dreams about joyful life events can represent opportunities for renewal and growth, while dreams about death tend to reflect unconscious anger or frustration, and may represent a wish to move on.

ARCHETYPES

Birthdays and Weddings, page 47

Pregnancy and Baptism, page 48

Baby, page 49

Killing and Drowning, page 50

Death and Burial, page 51

ASSOCIATED CARDS

○ Wedding

○ Baby

○ Killing

○ Drowning

BIRTHDAYS AND WEDDINGS

Dreams about birthdays usually reflect optimism about the future and satisfaction with the dreamer's current state of affairs. They may also be tinged with worry or linked with fears about aging and time speeding by. Wedding dreams reflect the coming together of the male and female parts of the psyche. They may relate to your marriage vows, express a wish fulfillment, or represent some other kind of emotional union.

GIFTS FOR THE FUTURE Opening birthday presents in a dream can signify feelings of excitement and curiosity about the future. Think how you felt about the presents; these emotions may describe your true feelings about the gift-givers.

GOOD LUCK MESSAGE Birthday dreams often portend good luck, especially in financial or work matters. Dreaming of someone else's birthday may signify your hope that good fortune will befall that person.

MISSED BIRTHDAYS A dream that your birthday was forgotten may indicate a fear of loneliness or a sense of being undervalued and not fully respected at work or at home.

CAKE AND CANDLES A dream birthday cake can demonstrate your willingness to share your life with others or to be generous with time or material objects. Candles indicate an optimistic outlook. But too many may also be linked with fears of aging and uncertainty about the future.

WHITE WEDDING A bride in white may reveal your moral attitude—toward sex, for example. In Western tradition, white represents purity, innocence, peace, and happiness, but in parts of the East white symbolizes mourning. If the bride was wearing a color, note its associations for you.

LADY-IN-WAITING? If you were a bridesmaid, how did you feel about the bride? Were you pleased for her—or jealous? Did you play an active part in the wedding, or did you hide from the conviviality? Did you catch the bride's bouquet?

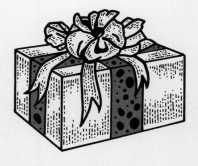

PREGNANCY AND BAPTISM

Dreams about pregnancy are associated with creativity and sustaining a new idea or project. Jung saw them as symbolizing the beginning of a new phase of personal development. The principal messages of baptism are rebirth, renewal, and resurrection. Such dreams usually mark the end of a stage in your emotional or physical life, and the beginning of a new one.

EXPRESSING A REAL DESIRE A dream of giving birth may simply be a form of wish fulfillment. Many women who wish for children report having had such a dream just before discovering that they are pregnant. Conversely, when a woman does not want a baby, such a dream may express fears of pregnancy, the pain of giving birth, or parenthood itself.

CARING NATURE For both men and women, a pregnancy dream can indicate a desire to nurture and care for someone else.

A FRIEND'S PREGNANCY Dreaming that a friend is pregnant indicates a deep wish for her to have a long and healthy life, and suggests a close bond between the two of you.

MULTIPLE PREGNANCIES Dreams that involve more than one baby may indicate divided loyalties. They warn you to weigh your priorities carefully, instead of trying to satisfy everybody at once.

PAINFUL PREGNANCY A painful or uncomfortable pregnancy is often connected with the demands of someone who is dependent on you. Perhaps you should consider ways of easing this burden.

NEW PROJECT A baptism dream strongly suggests immersion in a new project. Or, you may be working on an initiative that will prove successful. If your dream has any negative associations, future unforeseen circumstances may bring disappointment in their wake, but you will soon find a way to get back on track.

✎ A SYMBOL OF NEW STRENGTH Baptism rituals in real life symbolize rebirth and a commitment to a specific spiritual path. In dreams, they can indicate a desire to become stronger and more assertive.

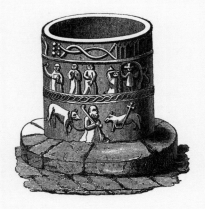

BABY

Many expectant mothers, or those planning to conceive, have vivid dreams about pregnancy, birth, and newborn infants. But for both women and men, baby dreams frequently illustrate other new beginnings, growth, or thoughts of nurturing. Does your dream baby represent you or someone else? If the baby is you, this may indicate a vulnerability and desire to be cared for.

BACK IN TIME If you are the dream baby, this may symbolize your original, innocent self, and can imply a desire to revert to such a state.

A CRAWLING OR WALKING BABY Seeing a crawling baby in your dream suggests the first stages in a new relationship or work situation. A walking baby signifies sudden independence. Seeing numerous babies can foretell the arrival of great happiness.

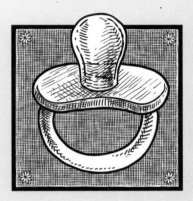

A TALKING BABY If you dream of a talking baby, this may indicate that you need to listen to your inner child—that your subconscious has an important message for you.

ROCKING A BABY Dreams about rocking a baby are usually linked with power. Such dreams can suggest that you are considering new work or family responsibilities, or may indicate a wish to better yourself. An attractive baby highlights prospective help from a friend.

FORGOTTEN CHILD A mother who forgets she has a child in a dream may be trying to hide certain weaknesses from others.

HUNGRY BABY A dream involving a hungry baby implies a desire for physical or spiritual nourishment. Baby dreams may also suggest that you have an unconscious longing for greater security.

BABY CRYING A dream of your own baby crying foretells positive news. A dream of someone else's crying baby may be warning you against taking on other people's problems, suggesting that perhaps it is time to start looking after yourself.

KILLING AND DROWNING

Whether you are murderer or victim, dreams about killing evoke strong, sometimes terrifying, emotions relating to power and vulnerability. Such dreams may express resentment, anger, or envy or may indicate an unwillingness to deal with some aspect of yourself. A dream of drowning suggests that you are struggling with real-life issues, or possibly that you feel overwhelmed by a female figure.

DEALING WITH ANGER If you dream of a massacre, ask whether you are angry with yourself, or if you feel enraged about some social injustice. Explore the strength of any anger you feel, and consider how to defuse it in your waking life.

☞ **UNDER ATTACK** A dream of being poisoned might relate to your vulnerability. Perhaps you feel that someone bears you a grudge and intends to deceive or attack you.

FIGHTING BACK Planning a murder in a dream may indicate that you are feeling intolerant of someone or something in your waking life. An accidental killing could be a sign that worries concerning social or work matters are unjustified. A killing carried out with a spear or a similar ancient weapon may be a sign of potential danger, or it may indicate a sense of dissatisfaction with some aspect of life.

MURDERING A RELATIVE Killing a family member could be linked with the idea of sacrifice. Such a dream may signify a need to give up something in order to achieve an aspiration in your waking life.

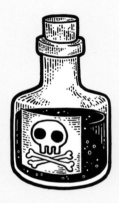

OVERWHELMED BY WAVES Dreams of drowning at sea can allude to feelings of insecurity and uncertainty about the future. Try to remember if land was in sight.

CALL TO ACTION While drowning dreams can indicate that you feel out of control, they may also be a helpful warning that urgent action is needed in your waking life to tackle immediate problems.

HERO OF THE HOUR Saving a drowning person in a dream may symbolize the fighter in you. Or, such a dream may suggest a cry for help from someone close to you.

DEATH AND BURIAL

Dreams of death or impending death can be terrifying but should not be taken literally. A dream of being buried alive, for instance, could simply be a graphic expression of feeling trapped. A funeral scene may be prompting you to examine your relationship with whoever is deceased in your dream, while a dream skeleton may suggest that you are reaching the heart of a complex issue.

☞ **LAID TO REST** The frightening dream prospect of being buried was traditionally seen as signaling difficult times ahead. While it often indicates a problematic situation from which you wish to break free, burial can also signify laying difficult matters to rest.

CURIOUSLY CELEBRATORY Strange as it may seem, a funeral dream can be a sign of upcoming celebrations. Dreaming of your own funeral indicates an end to a specific worry.

SAD OCCASION If you have fallen out with the deceased, the dream may express enduring hostility. If you felt sad in the dream, you may need to examine your feelings toward the deceased, and perhaps re-evaluate your behavior toward that person.

DYING FRIENDSHIP An empty black coffin can represent a lost friendship—although not through death. You may be worried that without a great deal of mutual effort a friendship cannot be sustained or revived.

PARENTAL FEELINGS A dream in which your parents die implies feelings of hostility toward them.

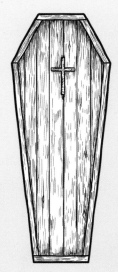

SKELETON DREAMS A positive skeleton dream may signal that you have analyzed and resolved a tricky problem. Unhappy dreams about skeletons suggest concern about a domestic issue.

MUSEUM BONES The appearance of a clinical skeleton in a dream, or of skeletons on display in a museum, is thought to indicate the arrival of new friends or colleagues in your life.

DREAM SETTINGS

The backdrop to our dreams may seem familiar but can also be symbolic; buildings can represent our very being. Dreams that feature natural surroundings often reflect a life path, indicating a potential for healthy growth or anxiety about emotional strength or spirituality. Vivid and dramatic dreams that focus on the fundamental forces of nature are traditionally linked with strong emotions.

ARCHETYPES	ASSOCIATED CARDS
The House, page 53	○ House
Places You Know, page 54	○ Tree
Castle or Place of Worship, page 55	○ Flowers
Trees and Green Spaces, page 56	○ Fruit
Branches, Leaves, Flowers, and Fruit, page 57	○ Ocean
Islands, Beaches, Mountains, and Rivers, page 58	○ Thunder
Oceans and Ice, page 59	○ Earthquake
Thunder, Lightning, Hail, and Storms, page 60	○ Fire
Earthquakes, Volcanoes, and Fire, page 61	○ Sun
Sun and Sky, page 62	○ Sky
Moon, Stars, and Planets, page 63	○ Moon

THE HOUSE

Whether familiar or unknown, exploring a dream house can signal the start of a journey of self-discovery, prompting you to develop some new facet of yourself. Discovering a new room in your own house suggests you may uncover a new aspect of your personality, or it could foretell imminent change. A dream of a childhood house can express a yearning for the simpler years of your youth.

DIFFERENT LEVELS A dream bungalow might suggest your life is currently being lived on just one level, practically or emotionally. A many-storied apartment building can imply that too much is happening in your life, and you need to focus on fewer areas.

UPSTAIRS, DOWNSTAIRS The attic of a dream house is thought to represent the dreamer's intellect and may signify new complex or long-term plans. Stairways are thought to portray success and progress, and can highlight ambition at work or in your personal life. Descending or ascending them may have sexual connotations. The basement or cellar of a house is said to represent those hidden crevices of the mind where fears and memories are buried.

BLOCKED DOORS OR WINDOWS Impassable doors or windows highlight feelings of frustration. Such dreams may be prompting you to stand up for yourself or for something dear to you. Blocked windows can represent an inability to see something for yourself; you may need to search further to uncover what you seek.

BRAND NEW HOUSE A new house is thought to symbolize your social life. If furnished, it may foretell a busy period of socializing, while an unfurnished house may signify a desire to extend your circle of friends.

🐚 **CAMPER OR TRAILER HOME** Dreams of living in a camper or trailer home may suggest that it is time to move on in some aspect of your life, and that failure to do so will lead to emotional stagnation.

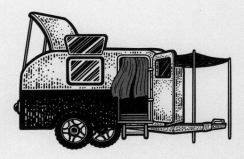

PLACES YOU KNOW

Familiar places, such as your home or neighborhood, frequently appear in dreams and can be a source of comfort when you are living far away from them and perhaps feel homesick. If you dream of a workplace, look for connections between the scene and your waking life; your emotions as you dream can be significant. Was the atmosphere tense, or was there a mood of purposeful creativity?

HAPPY WITH WHAT YOU KNOW?
Dreams of a familiar place often represent satisfaction with the past and contentment with the present. But if your dream is tinged with darker thoughts, the sight of familiar places may highlight dissatisfaction with a current situation.

LEARNING FROM EXPERIENCE Your
reaction to the familiar place in your dream may reveal whether or not you have learned significant lessons from your own life story.

LINK TO LOVE Dreams of being in your own office may predict a potential positive change in your love life.

SENSE OF LOSS Dreaming that you are excluded professionally, or have been ejected from your office, can denote a loss of property or of personal possessions.

LOCKED OUT A closed office can signify that something important is missing from your life.

TOO MANY PEOPLE An overcrowded office suggests feelings of being overwhelmed by excessive demands, while dreams of office problems may signal a fear of strife entering your life.

OFFICE TENSIONS The workplace is often associated with productivity and bustle, but it can also be a place of chores and intimidation. Offices encompass a great deal of physical and emotional energy. Were you content or stressed in the dream office? Your feelings may have implications for your life at work and at home.

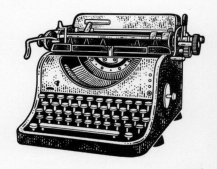

CASTLE OR PLACE OF WORSHIP

Dream castles tend to be associated with defense and attack, and can be a metaphor for such in personal or worldly matters. Note whether the castle was the launch pad for an attack, or if it was besieged by enemies. A dream place of worship is frequently associated with sanctuary and spiritual safety. Such a dream may also indicate a desire for some form of higher guidance in the dreamer's life.

WELL OR POORLY MAINTAINED Dreams of beautiful castles symbolize the prospect of a comfortable future, and the possibility that noble deeds will be performed. A castle in disrepair can warn of financial obstacles.

☛ **RELIGIOUS PLACE** Seeing a temple or other religious building in your dream indicates that moral issues may be at the forefront of your mind. You may be facing an ethical dilemma for which you are seeking guidance.

YOUR CASTLE, YOURSELF Castles, like other dream buildings, can represent you. Was the castle ornate, or was it still being built? Relate your answer to your personal strengths and weaknesses.

EARLY LIFE If the castle in your dreams resembled your childhood home, it may offer clues to how you felt as you grew up there.

LACK OF SPACE A cramped castle may indicate feelings of frustration and a lack of opportunities. A castle under siege suggests vulnerability and fears of being attacked.

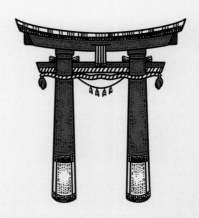

TEMPLE OF YOUR BEING In ancient times, a dream of a sacred building was thought to represent the dreamer's feelings of self-worth.

PEACE AND JOY Dreams of participating in a religious ritual can signify joy and contentment. Shunning a religious building or service can be a sign of guilt over a perceived wrongdoing.

BUILDING A PLACE OF WORSHIP Construction of a place of worship signifies the giving of presents to a loved one.

HOLY PERSON A priest or holy person usually represents someone you respect. Consider your feelings toward that person in the dream.

TREES AND GREEN SPACES

Dream trees have links to the deep unconscious. Their roots are associated with past events, and also with what lies beneath a person's visible exterior. A dream bush, like the biblical burning bush that the prophet Moses saw, may symbolize a desire for guidance, while dreaming of grass can be relevant to the outcome of future projects. For dream grass and parks, the level of maintenance may be key.

LOSS IN YOUR LIFE Chopping down a tree suggests memories or fears relating to the loss of a person or an object that you once held dear.

SCALING THE HEIGHTS Climbing a dream tree may express a desire to be honored. If a crowd was watching you climb, you may be seeking recognition.

THE HEALTH OF A DREAM BUSH A flourishing bush is usually linked with notions of support and may foretell the arrival of help from an unlikely source. A bush with little or no foliage can be a warning not to rely on good fortune alone in pursuit of a goal. Pruning a bush may be a sign that a secret will soon be revealed.

VERDANT OR DYING GRASS Green grass—especially near flowerbeds—can indicate success in work or leisure activities. Brown or dying grass can imply disappointment, or it may suggest that certain projects will be harder to achieve than originally thought.

CULTIVATED GRASS A dream of a well-tended lawn can pertain to an efficiently organized work project. Overgrown grass can signify stress in your waking life.

SEEDS OF SECURITY Planting dream grass is usually associated with the desire to provide security for yourself and your family. It can also suggest that your life will be enriched, but only in the long term.

A WALK IN THE PARK Dreams of strolling through a park with a loved one can signal good times ahead. Walking in a park with friends can symbolize divided loyalties. A poorly maintained park may foretell a period of readjustment and possible loneliness.

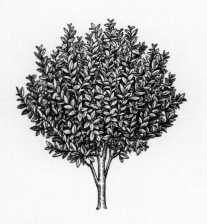

BRANCHES, LEAVES, FLOWERS, AND FRUIT

Traditionally, branches indicate good luck, growth, and new life. Healthy green leaves can symbolize growth and vitality, while dying or crumbling leaves may represent a lack of energy, or ending of an activity or project. The pleasurable, everyday association of flowers seems to carry over into dreams, making dreamers feel calm or reassured. Fruit traditionally symbolizes growth, the life cycle, sexuality, and fertility.

BRANCHING OUT Dreaming of swaying branches suggests that new activities or projects are ahead for you. They can also predict that life may soon take an interesting turn. Broken dream branches can signify concern about personal or work-related problems.

FLOURISHING LEAVES Leaves on a fruit tree can be seen as symbols of good financial luck or of prudent money management. The position of the leaves in relation to the tree in your dream can indicate how "contained" you feel in life. Those leaves growing close to a tree in a dream can symbolize personal satisfaction.

FLOWERS AND FORTUNES Dreams featuring everyday flowers may be connected to feelings of security in your career or home life. An abundance of flowers can foretell unexpected financial satisfaction. The sending of flowers is sometimes linked with personal satisfaction or the need for recognition.

ROSES, BUTTERCUPS, AND ORCHIDS Certain flowers have traditional connotations: the rose is associated with love and bravery, the buttercup with childhood, and the orchid with physical beauty and financial wealth.

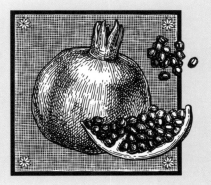

FRUITFUL DREAMS Eating dream fruit can have a sexual connotation. The luscious flavors can represent sensual enjoyment and sexual satisfaction. Certain fruits have links to parts of the anatomy: melons are said to symbolize breasts; peaches, the buttocks; and a banana, the penis.

PEACHES AND FIGS In many Asian cultures, the peach is a symbol of immortality, and peach blossom is linked with notions of femininity and female allure. In the West, the peach symbolizes redemption. The fig is universally viewed as representing fertility—an idea probably derived from its abundance of seeds.

ISLANDS, BEACHES, MOUNTAINS, AND RIVERS

In dream analysis, as in waking life, the desert island is an archetype of escape and isolation. A dream beach may seem a haven of tranquility or rather empty, possibly reflecting an attitude to leisure in waking life. Climbing a mountain or seeing a river in your dream may be linked with your journey through life.

ROMANCE OR REJECTION Dreams of a desert island may indicate that romance is coming your way. However, being cast up on a desert island can symbolize rejection or suggest a loss of self-esteem.

☞ **LONELINESS OR FREEDOM** A desert island dream may represent a yearning to escape the crowd or for loneliness to end. You may feel free—or marooned.

ESCAPE OR A GUARDED SECRET Dreaming of a beach can signify escape from your daily routine but can also suggest that you are keeping a secret from someone close to you.

TOP OF THE HEAP A dream of standing on top of a mountain is a sign of pride and honor. A quick ascent can represent the ease of your personal advancement.

HELP WITH THE CLIMB Did you climb your dream hill or mountain alone, or did someone help you? The answer could relate to how supported you feel in your waking life.

RIVER CROSSING Crossing a dream river in a vessel may represent a significant change in your life's direction. This can be interpreted positively if you are willing to embrace new developments in your waking life.

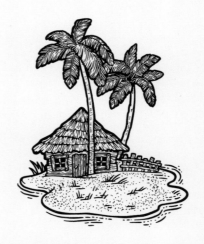

FLOW OF EMOTIONS A river can represent creativity and feelings. Observing it passively from the bank may indicate a need to get in touch with your emotions.

PLUNGING IN Falling into a dream river can be a warning of domestic concerns on the horizon. Jumping in may suggest that you should not take hasty action to resolve a pressing problem.

RIVERSIDE STROLL Walking along a riverbank can signify feelings of contentment with the progression of your career.

OCEANS AND ICE

In dreams, the ocean is often interpreted as signifying the unconscious, or as a symbol of motherhood or Mother Nature. It may also represent traditionally feminine characteristics, such as intuition. Dreams featuring water or ice can relate to the emotional parts of a dreamer's life as well. The transformation of water to ice can suggest the hardening of an emotion toward someone close to you.

OCEAN POWER In mythology, the dream ocean is a potent force; the strength of crashing waves echoes the human struggle on Earth. There is also a mystic tradition that the ocean is a form of "the one spirit" or a higher power.

VOYAGE TO FREEDOM A dream ocean voyage can predict a lucky escape in some domain of your life. The vessel you are sailing in may represent your home life—look for clues, such as the boat's name or color.

CALM WATERS The ocean may represent emotions, but also life in the womb. Floating calmly in warm water may be a "comfort" dream, a subconscious bid to reconnect with the environment of life before birth.

☞ **WRECKED FORTUNES?** A dream of being shipwrecked suggests fears of personal or financial ruin. How did you deal with the shipwreck? If you were part of a salvage team, what did you recover from the wreckage? If you took scant notice, consider whether you are trying to avoid a problem in your life.

BITTER COLD The perception of bitter cold in a dream usually represents an emotional extreme and may reflect an emotional numbness that you are currently experiencing.

HARVEST OMEN Ice dreams occurring outside of the winter season were traditionally thought to signal a fruitful harvest. A harvest can also represent the fruition of ideas, so consider which "crops" may need your attention.

MELTING ICE Dreams about melting ice can signal the unlocking of creative possibilities, foretelling that inspirational times may lie ahead at home or at work. It can also signify the thawing of a hostile relationship.

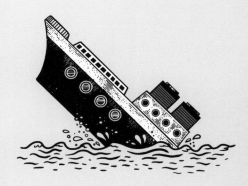

THUNDER, LIGHTNING, HAIL, AND STORMS

In ancient times, thunder and lightning dreams were associated with the voices of the gods, directing the dreamer with their power and wisdom. Today they are thought to suggest anger or to mark the conclusion of an episode in the dreamer's life. Cold, hard hailstones are associated with determination and perseverance, while storms are frequently interpreted as omens of imminent difficulties or danger.

DANGEROUSLY CLOSE Dream thunder that occurs directly above your home suggests that you are concerned about monetary loss or damage to your possessions.

NEWS FROM AFAR Hearing distant thunder may foretell that good news will arrive from a friend or relative in a distant country.

FALSE FRIENDS Muted thunder in a dream can signify that certain friends are not what they seem, and that they may have befriended you for ulterior motives.

CAUGHT IN HAIL Being trapped in a hailstorm can symbolize envy or jealousy. Enjoying the sensation of the falling icy stones may indicate that you relish a challenge. Escaping the storm suggests overcoming a succession of complicated hurdles.

POSITIVE CHANGES Dreaming about the end of a hailstorm can herald a positive change in your creative life. Such a dream may signify embarkation on a new project or a bold work-related initiative.

SHELTER AND ESCAPE Escaping a hailstorm may suggest that the dreamer can overcome complicated hurdles. Finding shelter from a dream storm can predict the positive resolution of a problem in your love life.

WAKING PROBLEMS A short-lived storm can denote smaller problems. A lasting tempest may reveal deeply rooted emotional difficulties.

⚡ POWER AND INSPIRATION Lightning dreams are usually connected to notions of power, inspiration, and strength. Consider how long the lightning lasted, and whether it made you fearful or exhilarated. Sudden flashes of lightning may signify a bright idea or insight.

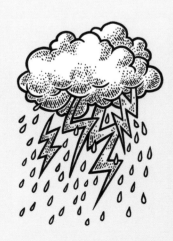

EARTHQUAKES, VOLCANOES, AND FIRE

Earthquake dreams often signify a perception that the world is in turmoil. They can reveal fears of instability, or concern that a major foundation of life is under threat. The tempestuous, fiery, and unpredictable nature of a volcano is usually associated with the eruption of suppressed emotions. Fire in dreams suggests destruction and purification, the severity and heat being direct representations of the dreamer's emotional being.

FALSE FRIENDS Hearing an earthquake's tremors and seeing its effects may signify that someone close to you could be trying to deceive you. If you witnessed your home shaking, the dream could indicate fears of instability in practical matters or in relationships.

FALLING MASONRY A building collapsing on you during an earthquake suggests that you are feeling the weight of your responsibilities.

SHIFTING PERCEPTIONS Volcano dreams can represent a massive shift in your internal world. They may signal the necessity of facing long-buried feelings or the realization that you must change your ways in order to progress on your life path.

SILENT WARNING A dormant volcano may be a warning about the reliability of new projects and a signal to consider all options before you act.

ERUPTING PROBLEMS A furiously erupting volcano can signify a potentially harmful situation of which you are unaware or have been ignoring. A smoking volcano can indicate a simmering passion.

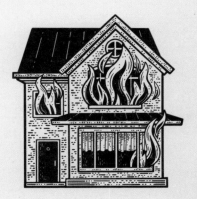

HOUSE ON FIRE A dream home on fire may represent you. The dream may be saying that you are in need of "cleansing," emotionally or physically. Were you able to stop the fire from spreading—or did it engulf the entire property?

SIGNIFYING HARDSHIP Dreams of crops in flames were traditionally interpreted as a sign of imminent famine or death. In a modern context, such dreams may signify lean times ahead.

LIGHTING A ROMANCE Building a fire—particularly if someone helps you—can presage a romantic alliance. Was your co-builder someone you knew, or a stranger? Were you able to contain the fire's flames together?

SUN AND SKY

Many analysts associate dreams featuring the sun with truth, power, and intellectual prowess. Its heat is usually linked with the emotional intensity of the dreamer's feelings and can also symbolize male energy. Across history the sky has represented an awesome presence beyond human reach. A dream sky is therefore often seen as symbolizing the height of what the dreamer wishes to achieve in real life.

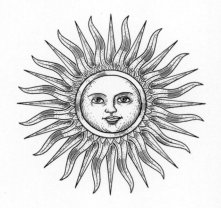

☞ **RISING SUN** A dream in which the sun rises majestically above the horizon can signify the advent of positive news. A rising sun can also represent the potential for the creation of wealth.

GOING DOWN A setting sun may symbolize a downward spiral in your life, and can foretell thwarted plans or ambitions.

RAYS IN THE BEDROOM Dreaming that the sun's rays bathe the bedroom in light is usually taken to signify financial gain.

SUN ON THE FACE A dream sun shining on your face or head is said to denote a sense of personal satisfaction. Such a dream may also signify the belief that others respect you.

UP IN THE SKY If you were flying in the dream sky, try to understand why you were doing so. For example, were you trying to get a bird's-eye view of a problem in your waking life?

BLUE SKY Some analysts believe that a very blue sky indicates that you will discover a lost or stolen item. It can also signify that a planned voyage will be successful.

PINKS AND BLUES A colorful sky is often linked with romance. It could symbolize a current relationship. It can also be a warning of an ill-advised tryst.

GRAY CLOUDS Dreams of cloudy skies can forecast turbulent times ahead. They may also signify that you are living "under a cloud," meaning that you are carrying some sort of weighty burden.

MOON, STARS, AND PLANETS

The moon governs the ebb and flow of the tides. In dreams it is associated with menstruation and even birth. It is thought to symbolize fertility, growth, and empowerment. Dreams of stars typically represent ambition and achievement. Planet dreams are often taken to mean that the dreamer is looking for some means of escape from their present earthly situation.

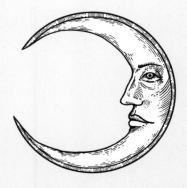

STARRY, STARRY NIGHT A dream of a clear sky filled with stars is generally viewed as a sign of prosperous times ahead or a possible future journey. Star dreams can also reflect the desire to reach unattained goals.

GUIDING LIGHT Your nearness to a dream star may indicate how close you are to realizing your ambitions. The dream star could be your "guiding light."

PALE AND WAN A sky filled with pale stars can signify difficult times ahead.

MOON PROMISE A dream moon is an optimistic sign, foretelling happy events. In aboriginal tradition the moon is believed to help women conceive.

A KINDLY MOON A dream moon shining onto your bed can signify forgiveness—either from you or to you. If the dream bedroom window is open, forgiveness may come quickly.

BRIGHT MOONLIGHT To dream of a bright moon may suggest that you will soon receive a financial windfall.

SPACE ODYSSEY A dream of flying to the planets may reveal an underlying sense of dissatisfaction with your daily routine and could signify an imminent life change—at work or in social or family affairs. Consider the ease or difficulty of the journey.

MARS, MERCURY, AND VENUS Dreams featuring Mars, the Roman god of war, are often associated with boldness, power, and the ability to achieve one's goals. A dream about Mercury, the Roman messenger of the gods, may be interpreted as a direct message from your inner self. Dreams about Venus, the Roman goddess of love, may reflect sexual desires.

DREAM CREATURES

Just like the animals of myths and legend, the creatures in our dreams have long been endowed with rich symbolic meanings. Sigmund Freud claimed that they often represent authority figures, including our parents. Dream animals may also be linked with some primitive instinct or "inner beast" that resides within the dreamer, but is repressed in waking life.

ARCHETYPES

ASSOCIATED CARDS

○ Bird

○ Wolf

○ Snake

○ Lion

BIRDS

In many mythologies the bird symbolizes both the soul and the conscious mind, and is also linked with spiritualism and shamans. Flying above the human world, the bird could contact the gods and form a connection between Earth and the heavens. In a dream context, this could signify the dreamer's unconscious relaying an important message or solution to a problem.

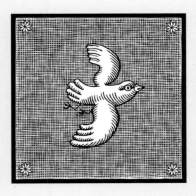

HEALING WINGS A bird in a dream may symbolize some aspect of the dreamer's inner world that can bring healing and wholeness. Bird dreams often leave the dreamer with feelings of exhilaration or empowerment.

A BID FOR FREEDOM Dream birds in flight can allude to a desire for escape. If the bird cannot fly, you may be feeling trapped in a difficult or demanding situation. A broken or clipped wing may denote that something is holding you back or blocking your path.

AN ALBATROSS, PEACOCK, OR SWAN An albatross in a dream foretells a weighty burden in need of immediate attention. A peacock is a sign of pride and satisfaction; its colorful and majestic plumage parades a personal achievement. The grace of a swan can allude to your ability to accomplish tasks smoothly and efficiently.

WOUNDED BIRD An injured bird in a dream portends worries, but not lasting ones. If you tend to a wounded bird, this may be a sign that the generous, caring side of your personality is currently active. If the injured bird is left to fend for itself, the dream may suggest that you are neglecting the kinder aspects of your nature.

SWEET SONGSTER A nightingale is often interpreted as a positive omen, signaling future success or possible financial gain. If a nightingale appears in your dream when you are ill, this can suggest that a quick recovery will follow. If the nightingale is singing, you may soon receive a promotion at work.

CAT AND DOG

Commonly seen as signifying wisdom, cunning, and good luck, cats are also associated with the mystery of life, death, and rebirth. Cats in dreams are linked with fertility and the prospect of new beginnings; they may also foretell personal or monetary good luck. Some believe that dogs in dreams suggest positive canine traits in the dreamer such as devotion, loyalty, and friendship.

YOUR CAT RELATIONSHIP The meanings of cat dreams may depend on your waking relationship with the animals. If you are afraid of cats, a dream cat may symbolize fears about aspects of yourself; if you love cats, a dream cat may reflect personal strengths.

BAD LUCK A cat that is killed or chased away in a dream may be construed as an omen of potential bad luck. A scratching cat can symbolize the desire to defend your territory, especially if you are feeling threatened.

MEOWING CAT A meowing or screeching cat is often thought to be a sign that someone is talking about you behind your back. Such a dream may highlight feelings of insecurity about friends or work colleagues.

NINE LIVES A cat that has one or more narrow escapes may suggest you will overcome multiple obstacles. The resilience of this "survivalist" cat may represent your own inner strength and tenacity in the face of adversity.

FRIGHTENING DOGS As with cats, if dogs frighten you in waking life, so will a dream dog. Aggressive dogs suggest fear of attack, possibly from a colleague or social acquaintance. Dog-lovers who have a frightening dog dream may be feeling vulnerable.

BARKING DOG A dream dog barking with excitement can express the feeling that you are socially accepted. A fiercely barking dog, however, may warn of potential work-related challenges ahead.

⚡ **MAN'S BEST FRIEND** A dream dog may represent a friend or acquaintance. A large dog may symbolize a soulmate or loyal friend. A small dog suggests concerns that your friendships are insignificant.

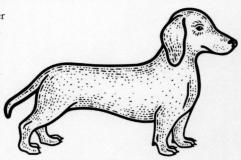

HORSE AND BULL

Dream horses can symbolize movement, freedom, and strength that could help us ride away in new directions. The horse is also said to represent the unconscious and, in certain mythologies, can speak in a human voice. The aggression and strength of a bull are often associated with masculinity. Dreams about bulls may express an innate desire to discover the masculine aspects of the self—or to avoid them.

CONTROLLING YOUR MOUNT A horse dream may indicate concerns or confidence in waking life. Note whether you were grasping the reins in fear or masterfully controlling the animal. A tethered horse can represent a part of you that needs to be liberated.

MOUNTING OR GALLOPING A rider mounting a horse in a dream may suggest potential prosperity. Galloping or racing horses are portents of speedy success at work. They can also denote feelings of elation, or the need to "ride above" the minutiae of the daily routine.

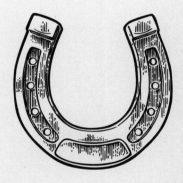

ANGRY HORSE A bucking horse warns of possible resistance to your plans and may indicate that you should spend more time persuading others. Dreaming of fighting horses implies tension among a group of friends.

TETHERED BULL Bull dreams often focus on tethering the creature. The ability to do so may convey how well you can integrate the "animal" aspects of your personality. Jung believed that the bull represented a person's true nature, and that the concomitant animal instincts were hidden behind multiple layers of consciousness.

GOOD LUCK Horseshoe dreams are often associated with good fortune. Grooming a horse may indicate the potential for luck in a speculative venture.

BULLFIGHTING Two bulls fighting can reveal disharmony among siblings—whether declared or underlying. Consider your position in the fight, and whether you were able to influence the outcome. A bull fighting a human may forecast the need for action to resolve an annoying facet of your personal life.

MOUSE AND RABBIT

Mice are generally thought to be timid creatures, although in cartoons they can be devious or cunning. Whether your dream mouse was hunter or prey may be an indication of your emotional strength. Rabbits are associated with fertility and sexuality. Like other fertility symbols, the rabbits of dreams are often interpreted as harbingers of personal growth and development, or as portents of a new project.

LUCKY RODENT Dreaming about a mouse may mean that you will receive some good or promising news shortly. A dream mouse or mice in the home may also signify prosperity as, in the past, a household with stored food was always an affluent one.

WHITE MISCHIEF Dreaming of white mice is commonly thought to indicate discord in your family or among your friends. If the dream mice are gnawing at food in your house, this may suggest concerns and irritations that require your attention.

ONE POSITIVE RABBIT A single dream rabbit can symbolize responsibilities that you will be happy to take on. A white rabbit can represent faithfulness in love.

RELISHING RABBIT A dream that centers on the eating of a rabbit can signify that you will enjoy your work and succeed at it.

LOTS OF RABBITS Seeing many rabbits in a dream can represent fears about potential enemies at work or in your social circle who may try to undermine you. In some interpretations, happy, frolicking rabbits are a more positive sign of fertility and a large family.

TIMIDITY AND EMBARRASSMENT
The overriding feelings associated with mice are timidity, embarrassment, and powerlessness. A mouse dream can therefore reflect a quest for increased emotional strength.

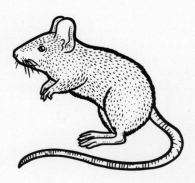

FOX AND WOLF

Cunning is the trait most commonly associated with foxes. Their appearance in dreams can be a signal from the unconscious to address this aspect of your personality, or the dream fox may represent a sly character in your waking life. The wolf has an equally deceptive, manipulative, and also potentially cruel image, and could similarly represent a facet of the dreamer or someone feared in waking life.

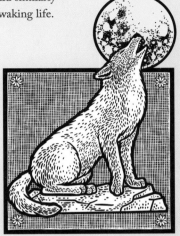

WARNING DREAMS Fox dreams are seen as harbingers of danger—especially hidden danger. Such a dream may alert you to be on your guard. Chasing, capturing, or killing a fox in a dream can signify plans to outwit those who may be plotting against you.

TAME OR WILD A fox in your home environment can indicate relationship difficulties. A fox that is seen in the distance may point to a betrayal of confidence.

FOX HUNTING A dream of riders hunting a fox may foretell an upcoming social event, or an enjoyable interaction with others.

FOX CUBS Dream fox cubs are thought to represent the warmth and coziness of the home.

MENACING PACK The sight of many wolves running together in a menacing pack signifies a fear of being robbed or cheated. The sight of a wolf's head can foretell success at work.

WOLF FANGS AND HOWLING Wolf fangs can symbolize fears of the unknown or anxiety about the future. Being bitten by a dream wolf can suggest that harm may come from your adversaries. A howling wolf may signal a cry for help from a family member or a close friend.

FAIRYTALE WOLF The classic fairytale wolf, as depicted in *Little Red Riding Hood*, may foretell a deception, warning that vigilance is needed. In a woman's dream, a fairytale wolf can symbolize a fear of male sexuality.

DOLPHIN AND FISH

The appearance of dolphins in a dream suggests that their widely acknowledged traits—intelligence, communication skills, grace, and playfulness—are present in the dreamer's waking life. By contrast, fish may symbolize a deep level of unconsciousness, according to Jung, because they are cold-blooded and are ancient participants in Earth's evolutionary history. Fish dreams may therefore indicate deep-rooted but unacknowledged wishes and fears.

BRIGHT MIND The appearance of a dolphin in a dream could be a sign that your intellect is being exercised, and that you are meeting cerebral challenges successfully. Dolphin dreams may also suggest that you need to leave present unhappiness behind, and move swiftly on to new challenges.

KEEPING IN TOUCH Dreams of dolphins are often associated with communication—or the lack of it—in your life, and might relate to your unconscious self trying to connect with your conscious self.

LEAPING DOLPHINS Dolphins diving in and out of water may represent successful management of the different aspects of your life.

COLD WATER Dolphins swimming in cold water may signify the need to change the way you are presently handling a certain task or duty.

WARM WATER Dolphins swimming in warm water may be seen as a sign of contentment with your current situation.

SHOALS OF FISH Many fish in a dream can symbolize fertility, or that good fortune lies ahead. The fish may also represent some form of encounter with your true self. Think about how they were swimming and whether you were part of the shoal.

FISHING NET Dreaming of a fishing net may indicate a fear of being found out. Fishing can also symbolize the notion of catching repressed feelings and bringing them to the surface.

PROSPERITY, GREED, OR FAILURE In some myths, fish in clear water are portrayed as omens of financial well-being. Dream fish may also represent greed or the hankering after material possessions, possibly at the expense of the spiritual elements of life. Dead fish are often said to represent disappointments or failures.

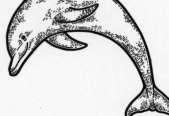

SNAKE, TIGER, AND LION

In the Judeo-Christian tradition, snakes symbolize evil. However, in Greco-Roman mythology, where the god of medicine carried a serpent-entwined staff, snakes are associated with healing. The power and cunning attributed to tigers may symbolize a person or situation that frightens or confuses the dreamer in waking life. Dreams about lions are most commonly linked with notions of bravery, pride, leadership, and protective rage.

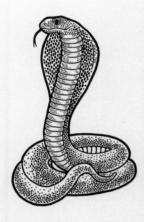

SNAKE DREAMS Snake dreams can highlight your innate wisdom or your sexuality. They can also signify a deep-rooted temptation or jealousy.

SELF-DEFENSE To dream of attacking or killing a snake is associated with overcoming those who wish to see you fail.

TIGER OMEN Dreaming of escape from a tiger is generally seen as a good omen, and may herald the arrival of positive news. However, dreaming of being chased or caught by a tiger in a dream can forecast danger in your waking life.

THE BEAST IN YOU The tiger is generally seen as a symbol of fear, but it may also represent the cunning or manipulative side of your personality.

LION DREAM Dreaming of a lion's ears was traditionally thought to highlight fears that someone close to you is envious. A lion's head in a dream can indicate that certain ambitions will be realized.

ROARING OR PLAYFUL A lion roaring aggressively may suggest the need to deal with the jealousy of a friend or deceit at work. A playful lion cub can predict new and satisfying friendships.

LION PRIDE A dream featuring a pride of lions indicates the possible start of a project in which you will lead or work closely with a team.

HOPEFUL FEMALE A dream lioness is generally seen as a sign of hope, particularly if she is protecting or lying down with her cubs. A lioness with her cubs may also symbolize positive family relationships.

EVERYDAY LIFE

Dreams about everyday actions and situations tend to relate to personal experiences. Your emotional reaction to them can reflect your feelings toward real relationships and the direction your life is taking. Dream travel, too, is usually linked with the dreamer's path through life. Everyday items in your dreams may be a reflection of recent events, but these familiar objects often have symbolic connotations.

ARCHETYPES

ASSOCIATED CARDS

○ Chasing

○ Climbing

○ Nakedness

○ Luggage

○ Missing a Ride

○ Automobile

○ Highways and Roads

○ Money

○ Jewelry

○ Food and Drink

CHASING, CHASED, AND CLIMBING

Whether you are pursuer or prey, a dream of being chased is likely to represent fear—of something in the real world or, more often, in the unconscious. Climbing is often associated with struggle—and ultimate success, if the summit is attained. Going up a mountain, in particular, can be seen as a form of escapism, indulging a wish to run away from part or all of your current life.

SINGLE PURSUER Being chased by one person in a dream is said to indicate a fear of intimacy in relationships.

MANY PURSUERS Being chased by a group may signify fears of being overwhelmed by work colleagues or family members, or of not having a say in some vital matter. It is sometimes associated with a missed deadline, unfinished work, or some sort of threat.

UNSEEN PREY Chasing unseen prey in a dream reveals directionless movement, and may suggest the need to clarify personal goals.

☞ **STAIRWAY TO SUCCESS** Climbing dreams can be symbolic of your current prosperity, achievement, and sense of personal fulfillment. Ascending a staircase or ladder signifies the pursuit of honor and respect. Or the steps may represent connections between different aspects of the self.

YOUR CLIMBING SKILLS Climbing a tree similarly implies ascending to a position of authority. Consider how quickly or slowly you were climbing, and how you felt if, and when, you eventually reached the top.

WALL DREAMS Scaling a wall denotes the need to find a solution—or some "sure footing"—with regard to a problem that may not yet be consciously recognized.

STARING INTO THE DEPTHS The existence of an abyss below you as you climb may mean that you are currently encountering a period of uncertainty or concern in your waking life. Such a dream may also refer to some form of personal journey that you are undertaking; the implication is that the journey is not over yet.

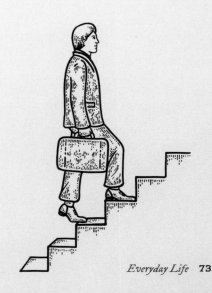

BEING NAKED

Naked dream images are associated with life's beginnings and the innocence of early childhood, and may represent a desire to go back to that state. The biblical story of Adam and Eve describes their unashamed joy before they obtained knowledge and saw the world's complexities. Their story is echoed in the personal desire to return to an infant past untrammeled by adult realities.

UNCOVERING THE TRUTH Dreams featuring nudity signify the desire to get beyond superficiality in personal relationships. Such dreams tell of yearnings to discover the "naked truth" about what makes a person tick.

HAPPY IN YOUR SKIN If the dreamer was naked in the dream and felt comfortable without any clothes on, this can imply a sense of personal ease and confidence in waking life.

EMBARRASSED BY NUDITY Shame at being naked in a dream can be interpreted as a fear of being exposed or humiliated. This can reflect your vulnerability or feelings of shame. A naked dream can also signify your fear about being caught off guard.

NO ONE NOTICES Sometimes in a dream you are shocked to find yourself suddenly naked, but no one around you comments or seems remotely concerned. This could signify that fears about your competence, or any other aspect of yourself or work, are unfounded.

FLAGRANT EXHIBITIONISM If you were flaunting your nudity in the dream, this may highlight a desire for new sexual encounters.

OTHER NAKED BODIES Dreaming of others taking their clothes off and parading naked may imply that members of your inner circle are deceiving you in some way.

REVEALING ALL If you have been accused and then cleared of a wrongdoing in the waking world, and you know that the charges were groundless, a naked dream may be your unconscious symbolizing elation at the outcome.

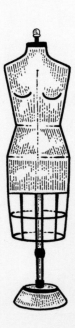

WASHING, BATHING, AND SEX

A dream that involves washing and bathing, both of which are often associated with spiritual cleansing, may be a bid to dispose of old or unwanted feelings or attitudes. A dream of sexual symbols may represent the union between a person's male and female energies. The sexual act itself may reflect the joining of the complementary but contrasting conscious and unconscious sides of the self.

DIRTY WATER If the water the dreamer bathed in was dirty, this can imply that he or she is currently in the process of spiritual or emotional cleansing.

FACE-CLEANING Washing the face in a dream is sometimes linked with the ending of a dispute or long-standing argument.

HAIR-WASHING A dream about washing hair is thought to denote the ability to avoid potential danger.

FOOT-BATHING While in waking life, bathing feet can be a ritual or a bid to relieve aches and pains, in dreams it is perceived as symbolic of unhappiness or dissatisfaction.

WISH FULFILLMENT Sexual dreams are often simple reflections of sexual desire or of past positive sexual encounters.

UNSATISFIED DESIRES Dreams that portray uninhibited sex may indicate that your real sex life is somehow stifled, while sexual teasing may symbolize unfulfilled ambitions.

UNINHIBITED PLEASURE Dreams of having sex in an unusual location can reflect a sense of exhibitionism or openness in you.

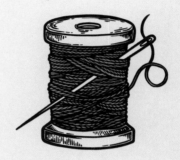

SEXUAL SYMBOLS In dreams, certain tools may symbolize sex. A hammer driving in a nail has been linked with sexual intercourse, while a dream needle and thread are thought to symbolize early sexual experiences.

NEW EXPERIENCES Dream participation in sexual acts that you have never experienced suggests a possible desire for experimentation in your waking life.

DREAM RING Dreams involving rings are often linked with the dreamer's sexuality. The dream ring may imply that your sexual nature is not entirely fulfilled at present.

SURGERY AND EXAMS

Dreaming about surgery is usually thought to foretell change. Such dreams are often frightening, but they can also contain motivational messages. More literally, they may signal the need to repair an area of your waking life. Exams are hurdles that must be overcome in order to reach a new stage. Success or failure in dream exams may reflect your inner thoughts about whether a problem can be resolved.

GOOD OMENS Operations in dreams can be harbingers of success or good news but may also reflect the need to overcome an obstacle.

☞ TACKLING PROBLEMS Dreaming of surgery indicates that you are considering changes in your life. The operation is a metaphor for the spiritual or emotional repair work that you need to do.

HEART, THROAT, OR NECK SURGERY A dream of heart surgery indicates that your emotions need your attention. A throat operation may be connected to the need for improved channels of communications. Operations involving the neck are linked with themes of flexibility and the need to be adaptable in relationships and work matters.

ENJOYING SUCCESS Dreaming about the diploma you receive for passing an exam reveals both your ambition and pride in what you do.

PASS OR FAIL Dreams of passing an exam with ease often presage or reflect positive achievements in real life, while failing in your dreams may imply a present inability to match your ambitions. Recurring exam dreams are common, and may represent judgments about succeeding or faltering at different stages of life.

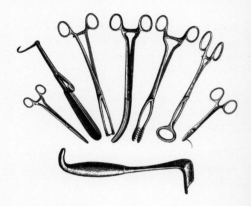

UNPREPARED FOR THE ORDEAL Exam dreams are typically linked with anxieties about being unprepared and to feelings of being tested in some way. Repeated exam dreams suggest feelings of failure.

WALKING OUT Leaving an exam early may indicate arrogance. Ask yourself if you displayed such behavior recently in your waking life.

GUILT TRIP Cheating in an exam can signify a sense of having attained something dishonestly in waking life.

BOAT, LUGGAGE, AND MISSED TRANSPORTATION

Many dream interpreters see the boat as a symbol of optimism and a sign that promising developments are just over the horizon. Dream luggage is often directly linked with emotional burdens and the need to shed them. Missing a means of transportation may simply reflect an actual fear of late arrival or the inability to meet a deadline, or it could relate to emotional strengths and weaknesses.

DENOTING CHANGE Dream boat trips, like other journeys, can be a hopeful indication of desirable transition or change. However, a rough trip may suggest a period of emotional turmoil. Were there calm seas ahead?

CALM WATERS Dreaming of sailing on a river, lake, or clear-water pond can signify happiness and success in your waking life. Walking on a boat can foretell future harmony and contentment. However, drifting suggests a deep-rooted fear of aimlessness in your personal life. It may also highlight worries that you are disorganized in a business matter.

PACKING AND UNPACKING A dream of placing objects inside a bag can express a desire to stock up on the good things in life. Unpacking a bag may be a sign of positive steps toward freeing yourself from a problematic relationship or an unrewarding job.

MISSING OUT Missed transportation may portray fears of missing a job opportunity or social engagement. An accidental delay could symbolize something in your life that you seek to blame for a misfortune.

CARELESS OR SUBCONSCIOUS WISH Missing your means of transportation may suggest a need to become more organized, or it may reflect an unconscious desire not to embark on a certain journey.

DREAM LUGGAGE A real journey, a change of relationship, or a new work venture are all possible interpretations of a dream about luggage. Luggage may also represent unexplored personal issues that weigh on your conscious or unconscious mind and emerge in the dream to encourage some form of resolution.

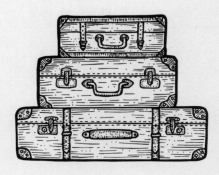

TRAVELING BY BUS, AUTOMOBILE, AIRPLANE, OR TRAIN

A dream journey by bus or car may indicate how you are negotiating your life. The route and whether you were passenger or driver can reflect its direction and whether you feel in control. An automobile may also represent you. Taking off in an airplane suggests both escape and the potential to launch a new venture. Depending on their movement, trains can symbolize security, elation, or postponement.

NO RESPONSIBILITIES Passenger dreams suggest freedom from responsibilities while someone else shoulders the burden. However, finding yourself in a crowd of passengers may indicate you feel hemmed in.

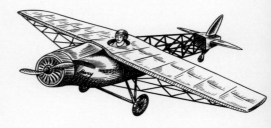

DRIVING A BUS Being the driver of your dream bus can show that you feel responsible for a group of friends or colleagues.

SMOOTH TRIP In a dream journey by car, the smoothness of the ride is thought to reflect your underlying emotions, while its speed can suggest how fast you are achieving your goals. The car is also considered a symbol of the male sexual organ or sexual powers in general.

DRIVING AMBITION Women's dreams of automobiles are often said to represent ambitious feelings and their desire to "overtake" the significant men in their lives.

REFLECTING LIFE Whether moving, stationary, delayed, or coming to a sudden halt, the progress of your dream train may directly reflect events in your waking life.

FLYING HIGH Piloting an airplane in a dream can represent an unexpected success in your life, perhaps in connection with work.

TAKE-OFF AND LANDING Taking off in a dream airplane may anticipate embarkation on a new project, while coming in to land may reveal that you are close to finalizing a work arrangement or personal matter.

TRAINS AND TUNNELS Like automobiles, dream trains are sometimes thought to symbolize the male organ. As entering a tunnel therefore represents coitus, consider how that makes you feel.

MONEY, JEWELRY, AND ENVELOPES

Most interpreters believe that money dreams express the ability to give and receive in emotional terms, but they can simply reflect the dreamer's generosity, greed, or other waking use of money. Dreams about jewelry are often connected with wish fulfillment. Sometimes, the jewels are viewed from a distance—possibly with envy or desire. Dream envelopes often symbolize a message that the dreamer anticipates or wishes to communicate.

BUSINESS INSIGHT Giving money away in a dream is generally seen as a good omen. Recall who was paid, how much they received, and why. The answers might shed light on current work-related issues.

INVESTING IN THE FUTURE A dream of saving or investing money may reflect your financial planning for the future. Or, it may imply that you have taken the necessary steps to prepare yourself emotionally for developments within certain relationships.

STRING OF PEARLS A dream of pearls around a woman's neck is usually seen as a positive sign, and can signify marriage or the possibility of children. Dream pearls may also relate to future transactions.

RARE JEWEL A dream of viewing a rare jewel that you do not own can mean that you will fail to understand the importance of a particular future friendship. Failure to accept this friendship may cause difficulties later in life.

FACETS OF FRIENDSHIP A diamond's many facets can imply the need to consider a relationship problem from a number of angles—or to examine the individual parts of it.

LOTS OF ENVELOPES A dream of many envelopes can suggest the expectation of news, or that new projects are on the horizon.

OPEN ENVELOPES Dreams of open envelopes may represent the onset of trivial problems that can easily be overcome. A tightly sealed envelope can signal a change of direction or emotional or practical obstacles ahead.

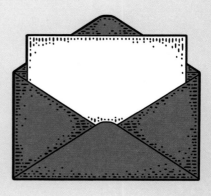

SHOPPING AND GARDENING

Dreams about shopping are important indicators of needs and desires. Extravagant buying suggests a quest for instant gratification, while a small purchase suggests a carefully reasoned approach in real life. The dream garden, too, often represents the dreamer. A lush green garden can symbolize internal growth and indicate a positive phase of life, while an overgrown plot may imply neglect of self or others.

FREEDOM AND CHOICE Shopping dreams are tied to notions of freedom, choice, and the ability to make unhindered decisions.

SHOPPING STYLE The way you shop in dreams may be significant. Hurried shopping can indicate a lack of self-restraint, especially in financial matters.

EMOTIONAL NEEDS Dreams of shopping may also be a direct reflection of your current emotional needs. Were you doing the week's shopping calmly, or were you stocking up in case of an emergency?

HIDDEN DESIRES Food shopping in a dream can express a hidden attempt to "buy" other people's attention or devotion. Dreams of shopping for items you want in real life may highlight the reality that you cannot always get what you desire.

MANAGING EXPECTATIONS A dream of owning or managing a store suggests feelings that people are too reliant on you.

☞ **GARDENING TRIUMPHS** Dreams involving gardens can signify future gain and financial success. The planting of seeds can symbolize the birth of new ideas.

WELL-KEPT OR ILL-KEMPT The garden's condition may reflect the current state of your psyche. Was it blooming or choked with weeds? Were the paths smooth or broken? Gardening in a dream can sometimes signify sadness.

CUTTING BACK Pruning roses or other plants may symbolize tension in personal relationships.

AUTUMN FRUITS An orchard in your dream can suggest that you are harvesting the fruits of your accumulated wisdom.

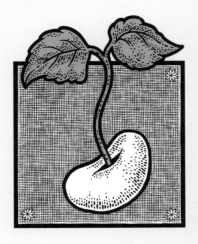

TOOLS, BROOMS, AND GARBAGE

Dreams featuring tools are sometimes interpreted as symbols of masculinity and male sexuality. With their potential for digging and concealing, tools may also represent elements that are locked away deep in the dreamer's memory. Dreams of brooms typically represent a desire to sweep away the past or current unwanted obligations. Dreams about garbage can signal the desire to jettison unwanted aspects of life.

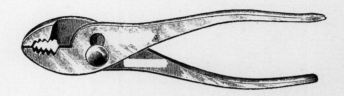

FUNCTION OF THE TOOL A tool's use may have some bearing on the dreamer's psychological state, expressing the need to clear, build, or renovate spiritually or mentally.

LIFTING UP A dream that focuses on lifting or leverage is generally interpreted as a wish for increased personal growth. Was the process difficult? If there was a problem, how was it ultimately overcome?

DIGGING DOWN As in waking life, dream spades can be used for digging and covering things over. If you were digging, what were you searching for? If an object was being concealed, was it associated with something that you might be trying to avoid?

NEW BROOMS In dreams, new brooms traditionally foretell good luck. They may suggest that good times lie ahead, and that chances should be seized. However, a damaged dream broom can reveal feelings of insecurity or suspicion of an acquaintance.

CHASING WITH A BROOM A dream of chasing someone with your dream broom could signify that a surprising change for the better is on the horizon.

COVERED IN GARBAGE A dream in which you were covered in garbage may imply that you feel overburdened in waking life. Note if and how you escaped—did someone help you or did you manage alone?

CHANCE DISCOVERY A valuable object in your dream garbage may foretell an unexpected piece of good news in the near future.

DISCARDED TREASURE If precious goods were unwittingly placed in the garbage, try to work out who put them there. Is there someone close to you who may be trying to spoil an event or project?

FOOD AND DRINK

Being so significant in waking life, it is hardly surprising that food and drink often feature in dreams. Both represent affection, appetite, or a desire to live life to the fullest. Biting or chewing in a dream may be connected with sensual pleasures, while overeating can suggest an emotional or practical overload. Meager portions may signal deprivation and the need for some form of "nourishment."

SELF-INDULGENCE Dreams of rich foods, such as creamy sauces and chocolate, are said to be signs of extravagance. Note how you felt while consuming the food. Did you feel guilty about the quality or the abundance of it, or did you feel justified in enjoying it?

CAUSE FOR CELEBRATION In dreams and reality, wine is associated with both pleasure and ritual—the celebration of weddings and births, for example. If the dream wine was consumed in company, you may be anticipating a joyous event, even if the occasion has not yet been officially acknowledged.

THE START OF SOMETHING Just as breakfast is the first meal of the day, the dream breakfast can mark the beginning of a new project or a new stage in your life. Was the food consumed at a leisurely pace, or was it rushed?

COMFORT FOODS Dreams about dairy products can be inner yearnings for things past. Symbolic of the nurturing bond between mother and child, milk in a dream can reflect dependency or a desire for emotional nourishment from someone close to you.

DINING OUT The atmosphere of your dream restaurant can reveal your emotional state. Wholesome or elegant surroundings indicate contentment with life, while a dimly lit establishment, where the service is poor and the food mediocre, may indicate a need for inspiration or some form of personal satisfaction currently missing from your life.

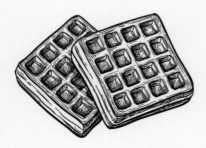

CUTLERY AND CONTAINERS

Dreams featuring cutlery are widely thought to represent the masculine and feminine aspects of the dreamer. A knife and fork together can also signify a balanced lifestyle, or they may represent emotional or personal growth. Dreams of containers, such as boxes and bags, can symbolize areas of the dreamer's psyche. Such dreams may allude to notions of security, safety, and containment—in an emotional or a real sense.

NOURISHING SPOON DREAMS Dreams of spoons can symbolize enduring domestic or familial happiness. Spoons that scoop up food can represent nourishment and may signify that life is good.

SMOOTH SHINING LIFE Dreaming of a shiny spoon can suggest a smooth home life. Similarly, a set of new spoons can indicate harmony within the family group.

GIFT KNIFE A dream of giving a knife as a present may be a warning that a project will be curtailed prematurely. Think about how you might circumvent this in your waking life.

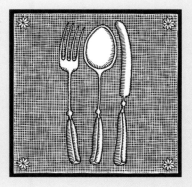

UNLOADING PROBLEMS A dream featuring heavy containers could be a signal that you need to unload some sort of burden; their contents are significant.

AN EMPTY DREAM An empty dream container may suggest that the dreamer's waking life needs to be filled, either emotionally or with new challenges.

SOMETHING MISSING An empty box in your dream may be telling you that something is missing from your life. Did you open the box to discover that it was empty—and were you surprised? Your reaction may reflect your present level of emotional satisfaction.

OVERFLOWING CONTAINERS Jars or pots can symbolize social gatherings, or a desire to expand your circle of friends. Overflowing jars or pots may suggest that you feel overwhelmed by emotional or personal issues.

KNIFE AND FORK A dream knife that appears rusty or broken can reflect fears of family strife or love-life problems. By contrast, a dream fork that is used to blend tasty ingredients can foretell busy and enjoyable social events in the near future.

DECODING COLORS

We interpret what we see in waking life—and also our dreams—in terms of both form and color. In both worlds, colors can have several meanings—for instance, white symbolizes purity in the West but death and mourning in the East. Yellow can suggest bright intellect or cowardice. In dreams, reality may also be curiously transformed, and ordinary things may be unusually colored—often reflecting the dreamer's mood or a powerful emotion.

ARCHETYPES

White, page 85

Pink, page 86

Red, page 87

Orange, page 88

Yellow, page 89

Green, page 90

Blue, page 91

Purple, page 92

Black, page 93

ASSOCIATED CARDS

○ King and Queen

○ Face

○ Tree

○ Flowers

○ Fruit

○ Fire

○ Sun

○ Sky

○ Bird

○ Money

○ Jewelry

○ Food and Drink

DREAMING IN WHITE

Because the color white has highly varying cultural connotations, your own background will dictate your reaction to the color. Its associations with mourning make it the color of sadness in the East. In a Western context, dreams featuring white can reflect feelings in the dreamer that are untarnished and pure. The appearance of white in a dream can also indicate that the dreamer's future is bright and uncomplicated.

ROYAL PERSON A white royal family member can be a symbol of hope. Consider whether an authority figure has recently offered you encouragement.

WHITE TREES A forest or woods filled with white trees can signify a desire to enter a new, positive phase of life.

PEACEFUL A white room can indicate a current state of tranquility.

PURE FOOD A cook or chef dressed in white may suggest that you need "pure" nourishment, love, and affection from those around you.

YOUR SPACE A white stage or podium can relate to success in public affairs.

QUIET ENCOURAGEMENT Dreaming of a white hand may symbolize a new or improving personal relationship.

PERSONAL SUCCESS White clothes suggest you will be successful in current undertakings.

SIGNALING A TRUCE A white bird—particularly a dove—symbolizes peace. In a dream, it may represent a desire to end personal or societal conflicts.

HONEST EFFORT A white flower in a dream can symbolize simplicity and purity in some aspect of your life.

SOLID FOUNDATIONS A white book may denote that you are laying the groundwork for a successful enterprise.

A DESIRE FOR CLEANSING White water can relate to purity and the need for cleansing in your emotional or personal life.

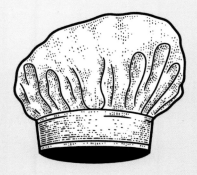

DREAMING IN PINK

In Western cultures, pink is the color of femininity and is also often used in confectionery and cakes to signify sweetness. It is thought to have a calming influence, and in the East can symbolize both marriage and trust. While light pink suggests innocence, a deeper pink may have sexual connotations. As the following common examples show, pink dreams are often associated with emotions.

WINDOW OF OPPORTUNITY The image of a pink window can represent a personal opportunity that has not yet been revealed.

NEW RELATIONSHIP Dreams of a pink cloth or mat may mean that you are considering entering into a new relationship or friendship, and are weighing up the implications.

SECRET PASSION A pink closet can signify that you are currently storing love for someone special, while waiting for the right moment to reveal your feelings.

LOOKING FOR LOVE Pink clothes can indicate a wish to be "covered" in love by someone close.

EMOTIONAL STABILITY A pink chair may signify emotional stability, especially if it remains unmoved during the dream.

SPECIAL AWARD A pink statue can be a sign of success in a work project.

REWARD FOR DILIGENCE Pink steps may suggest that you will accomplish a personal task through hard work.

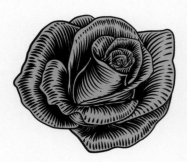

ROSY PROSPECTS Pink flowers are seen as symbols of future pleasurable activities.

BUSINESS HOPE A pink poster can be an indication of a potentially beneficial transaction in the near future.

DEEP EMOTIONS A pink figure or face may signify that you are in the process of revealing deep emotional feelings to someone in your waking life.

DISTANT LOVE A pink heart or heart shape could be related to pangs of love for someone who is far away.

DREAMING IN RED

With its connotations of fire, heat, and blood the color red is usually connected with energy, vitality, and anger. The appearance of the color red in a dream can suggest passion for a project or relationship in the dreamer's current life. Alternatively, it can denote unconscious feelings of rage toward a person or situation. It may be associated with a feature of the body, an emotion, or a force of nature. Here are the meanings of some the most common red dream symbols.

FIERCE PASSION A red heart can reveal deep-rooted passion or sexual energy that you are presently experiencing in waking life.

TROUBLING RASH A red rash tends to indicate feelings of irritation or embarrassment about a situation in waking life.

GOING RED Bright-red ears can point to sensations of guilt, shame, or embarrassment.

INQUISITIVE NOSE A red nose in your dream can refer to current feelings of curiosity, or perhaps to a "nosy" desire to delve into the affairs of others.

FIRE HAZARD Red flames in a dream can indicate a perception of imminent danger. It is important to take heed of such a warning.

RICH RED Red wine in a dream can denote richness, personal satisfaction, or happiness in your life.

LOSING A FRIEND Possibly because red has undertones of anger, red paper may be connected to the loss of a friendship.

BLUSHING BRIDE A red wedding dress, as worn by brides in the Hindu tradition, is believed to symbolize life itself.

SYMBOL OF LOVE A red rose can be a symbol of romance and eternal love.

☝ **MARK OF DISTINCTION** A red balloon can symbolize your uniqueness and the feeling that you stand out from the crowd.

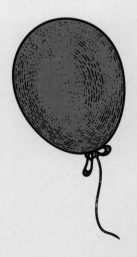

DREAMING IN ORANGE

Orange is commonly thought to symbolize nobility and generosity. It can also represent radiance, optimism, and tranquility. Dreams in which orange appears can therefore signify positive change in the dreamer's waking life; several travel-related dream symbols illustrate this. Some dream interpreters also contend, however, that the color orange suggests feelings of mistrust and doubt, and thus a dream in which it features may reveal discontent or uncertainty.

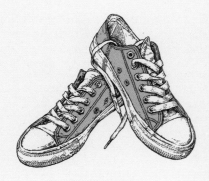

↳ **ON THE MOVE** Orange running shoes can represent positive movement toward a future destination. Their appearance may be tied to a current project on the verge of completion.

NEW HORIZONS An orange map or atlas may illustrate a desire to travel or to seek out new terrain, either practically or emotionally.

GOLDEN GROUND Orange soil denotes a positive journey—possibly in connection with work or work colleagues.

BITTER JOY Despite its unpleasant taste, a sour orange can be a sign of happiness.

LIFTING YOUR SPIRITS An orange elevator can denote an upturn in your emotional state following a depressed period.

BRIGHT HEADWEAR An orange hat in your dream can symbolize creativity or the dawning of a bright new idea.

ANGRY GESTURE An orange arm or fist can denote feelings of hostility or aggression.

BRIGHT AND FLOURISHING An orange flower can represent feelings of vitality and a general contentment with your life.

BURSTING WITH IDEAS An orange volcano can express a surge of creativity that is waiting to burst forth from you.

ORANGE YOU If you appear to have turned orange in your dream, this can be a sign of self-protection or of self-love.

SIGNALING A DELAY An orange road sign can denote that an expected change in your current situation could be delayed.

DREAMING IN YELLOW

According to some dream analysts, the color yellow represents the dreamer's intellect and degree of linear thought, and may be an indication of clear, decisive thinking in some sphere of his or her life. Yellow is also traditionally associated with fear and cowardice—hence terms such as "yellow belly." In the context of dream actions and situations, a number of symbols often appear in conjunction with the color yellow.

HITTING THE TARGET A dream of shooting yellow arrows or darts may indicate that you will reach your current goals by thinking clearly.

ACTIVE PLAYER OR TIMID OBSERVER If a yellow ball appears in a dream game, try to recall whether you contributed to the game—or whether you stood timidly on the sidelines.

FEELING LIKE AN OUTSIDER Playing in a dream playground of a yellow hue may be evocative of feelings of exclusion in your younger days.

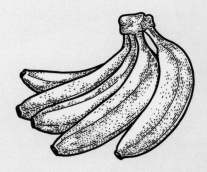

IN THE SPOTLIGHT Sitting in a yellow room may be a sign of heightened awareness of a particular situation. Try to determine what that situation is, and whether there is anything you can do to improve it.

EMBRYONIC THOUGHTS An egg yolk signifies notions of creativity and vitality.

BURNING BRIGHT A burning yellow sun can symbolize energy, strength, and the circle of life.

FOOD SYMBOLS Dreams about yellow foods, such as pineapple, bananas, or custard, can represent feelings of cowardice.

SIGNIFYING A SETBACK A yellow notice can be a sign that change will occur but that setbacks may interrupt its pace.

SICKLY PALLOR Murky yellow in a dream can reflect fears of sickness or failing health.

SIGN OF DECAY Yellowing, dying grass can be a signal that you are in need of physical or emotional nourishment.

DREAMING IN GREEN

Because of its close links to nature, some dream analysts associate the color green with feelings of calm, hope, growth, and sustenance—indicating the start of a flourishing period of personal growth or spiritual development. Green, however, also has negative connotations: it can denote jealousy, envy, and decay. Thus, a green dream may be a prompt to face up to such troubling feelings and to try to deal with them positively.

COMING TO FRUITION A greenhouse can indicate that hard work will bring a successful conclusion to your plans.

LONG LIFE An evergreen tree can symbolize longevity or immortality.

FULL OF GOODNESS Green vegetables, whether one or many, can denote growth, good health, and the advent of personal nourishment.

NOT YET MATURE Green fruits imply that a present project is not "ripe" and must be planned more carefully.

PEACEFUL SETTING A green field can represent an expanse of calm and equilibrium in your waking life. Green moss may also reflect feelings of peace and security.

EMOTIONAL WRECKAGE Green earthquake debris can signify envy in a close relationship.

ROTTING FLESH Green flesh can symbolize some form of rottenness or corruption.

YOUR GROWING SKILLS Green fingers can foretell a period of personal growth or creativity.

EYES OF ENVY Green dream eyes traditionally symbolize feelings of jealousy.

VALUABLE GEMS Green jewels or precious stones can relate to feelings of security and calmness, but may also reflect feelings of envy.

STAGNANT WATER Green water can reflect feelings of stagnation and may indicate the need to be proactive in your life.

A LONG WAY TO GO A green pathway can indicate a journey of considerable distance.

PAPER MONEY Green bank notes can refer to a current project that involves a transaction that is being carried out from a distance.

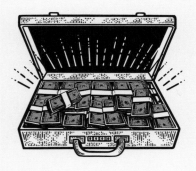

DREAMING IN BLUE

The color blue is thought to represent the power of the conscious mind—especially if it appears in a dream sky. It is also traditionally associated with transparency, spirituality, and infinity. Some analysts believe that the appearance of blue in a dream can indicate feelings of gentleness or patience. Different shades of blue can reflect the dreamer's present emotional state; a bright blue may suggest happiness, while a brooding indigo may foretell a downward emotional cycle.

EMOTIONAL HEALTH-CHECK Blue water is often linked with the dreamer's emotional life. Vivid blue dream water can be a sign that you need to pay attention to your emotions.

FEAR OR EXHILARATION Blue hail in a dream, like falling rain, usually has emotional significance. Try to recall how long the hail lasted. If you were caught in a hailstorm, did it make you feel afraid or exhilarated?

DESIRE FOR ESCAPE A dream featuring gusts of blue air can signify a yearning for freedom in your emotional or working life.

SWIRLING OR SCREENING If blue smoke appeared in your dream, did it obscure your view—or swirl toward a specific destination?

☞ **FREEDOM STONE** A blue gemstone can signify liberation from a current problem.

BOY'S COLOR Blue clothes can be a symbol of masculinity, or of the male side of your nature.

BIRD OF HAPPINESS A blue bird may symbolize happiness, hope, and liberation.

CLIPPED WINGS A caged blue bird can signal a lack of independence and a yearning for emotional freedom.

FEELING BLUE? Blue paintings or drawings in a dream may be general reflections of your present life circumstances.

BLUE HAZE A dream photograph tinted blue suggests that something is obscured from view in your waking life.

BAD FEELINGS A blue heart may refer to a quarrel between yourself and a loved one.

COLD AND CLOSED A blue vase can be a sign that you feel emotionally contained.

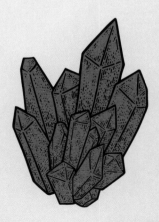

DREAMING IN PURPLE

The color purple traditionally symbolizes authority, majesty, and the law. In Western societies, the legal professions and the monarchy are typically adorned in shades of purple. The appearance of purple in a dream, therefore, is said to represent loyalty, truth, justice, and spiritual penitence. Some claim that the color also expresses the dreamer's current state of psychic awareness and can predict future happenings.

SIGNIFYING PERSONAL PRIDE A purple bird can be a symbol of pride, prowess, or personal dignity.

☞ **FREE-FLOWING SPIRITUALITY** Exotic purple fish swimming together in a dream can signify free-flowing spirituality.

POWERFUL FEELINGS The appearance of a purple leopard or cheetah in a dream may represent the strength of your emotions.

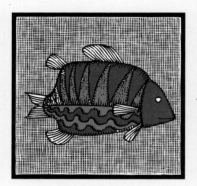

BEAST OF BURDEN A dream about a purple camel can signify excessive subservience to an authority figure.

SYMBOL OF CEREMONY A purple procession can foretell the advent of pomp and ceremony in your future.

UNSOLVED MYSTERY Purple crystal may indicate that there is an unsolved mystery in your current waking life.

SELF-AWARENESS A purple glass can represent your intuition or self-awareness.

INNER FIRE A purple flame can be a direct connection to your unconscious.

FESTIVE OCCASIONS People tinted purple appearing in a dream can foretell festive social occasions in your future.

PURPLE WARNING A purple pen may signify that you need to be more truthful in your communications.

LACK OF CONFIDENCE A purple book can suggest that you lack self-confidence.

DREAMING IN BLACK

In many cultures, black is a symbol of grief and mourning. Like the color blue, it is often linked with "dark" moods and can convey feelings of depression. Yet some dream analysts see black as a color of hope and believe that its appearance in a dream can bring highly positive messages. Black can also be seen as a symbol of the shadowy or unrealized part of the dreamer, suggesting unfulfilled potential.

FUNEREAL THOUGHTS Black in the context of a funeral may signal difficulties ahead. Try to recall if the dream hinted at their nature.

OMINOUS BIRD A magpie that features in a life-or-death scene is usually interpreted as a message that you will not succeed with a particular love interest or project if you continue to approach it from the same angle.

STRANGELY COMFORTING A black shroud or sheet can represent warmth, comfort, or a return to less complicated times.

SIGN OF A SETBACK Blackberries in a dream can be a sign of a setback on the way to the resolution of a particular goal.

CALL FOR COURAGE Blackbirds in flight can indicate that you will be required to demonstrate great practical or moral courage in the future.

FINANCIAL WARNING To dream of a blackboard with chalk marks on it can show concern about the security of your finances.

DEEP SUBCONSCIOUS A black hole or dark cellar can represent the workings of your unconscious mind.

GOING NOWHERE A very dark night can reveal a sense that your life lacks direction.

LUCKY IN LOVE A black necklace worn to a celebratory event may be a positive omen in the realm of romance.

BLACK SHEEP Dreams of black sheep are associated with temptation, envy, or greed.

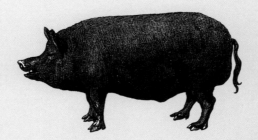 **REPRESSED FEELINGS** A black dream animal can be a symbol of repressed emotions or unfulfilled aspirations.

INDEX

About the Author

Dr. Fiona Starr is a clinical psychologist and principal lecturer
in clinical psychology. She is also a family counselor in
London, England, and a supervisor of psychology students.

PICTURE CREDITS

6, 67, 79 Shutterstock/MoreVector;
background 8–9, 16–17, 30–31
Shutterstock/Yuzach; 9 Shutterstock/
Tartila; 10 Shutterstock/Sentavio; 11,
22 Shutterstock/blue67sign; 12, 13,
14, 18, 24, 26, 38, 41, 42, 44, 47, 50, 53,
54, 55, 58, 59, 60, 61, 62, 63, 66, 68,
69, 70, 71, 73, 74, 75, 77, 80, 85, 87, 89,
90, 91 Shutterstock/Alexander_P; 15,
34 Shutterstock/Viktoriia_P; 17, 23
Shutterstock/Kseniya Parkhimchyk; 20
Shutterstock/bioraven; 21 Shutterstock/
ArtColibris; 28, 65, 83, 92 (plus background
42, 49, 57, 69, 80) Shutterstock/Bubica;
29, 56, 57, 82 Shutterstock/NataLima;
31, 45 Shutterstock/Channarong
Pherngjanda; 32, 39, 86 Shutterstock/
Christos Georghiou; 37 Shutterstock/
Babich Alexander; 40 Shutterstock/Maisei
Raman; 43 Shutterstock/Hein Nouwens;
48, 81 Shutterstock/Morphart Creation;
49, 51 Shutterstock/Bodor Tivadar; 76, 93
Shutterstock/lynea; 78 Shutterstock/Artur
Balytskyi; 88 Shutterstock/DianaFinch.